INTERMITTENT FASTING 16/8:

THE COMPLETE GUIDE TO THE INTERMITTENT FASTING DIET 16/8 FOR BEGINNERS, WOMEN, MEN AND OVER 50. PROMOTE HEALTH AND WEIGHT LOSS THROUGH AUTOPHAGY.

By

ROSANNE MILLER

Table of Contents

Introduction

Fasting doesn't cause bad health. Fasting does not cause death. Fasting is not dangerous. Cavemen and cavewomen fasted because of a lack of food and a need to preserve, many religious practices encourage fasting, such as the Muslim Holy month of Ramadan, and during Lent in Christianity. Put simply, fasting isn't something out of the ordinary, and the human body is more than capable of going without food for a short amount of time. Your body naturally fasts during your sleeping time at night!

Before we begin, you need to banish the idea that fasting is dangerous out of your mind. Fasting is safe, provided you follow the rules and eat when you're supposed to. There is a very big difference between fasting and starving. When you attempt to starve yourself, you're doing so because you are choosing not to eat. This is dangerous and comes with a myriad of serious health concerns attached to it.

Warning aside, let's delve a little deeper into the world of intermittent fasting and explain exactly what it is.

Intermittent fasting, as the name suggests, is fasting intermittently throughout the day. It is a cycle of eating and fasting, and the plus point is that there are no rules in terms of what you can eat and what you can't, provided you stick to health in general. For this reason, intermittent fasting is the eating pattern of choice. You can still enjoy the odd bar of chocolate if you want to, but you need to ensure you stick to moderation and that you do so within your eating window only.

Basically, intermittent fasting doesn't tell you what to eat, it tells you when to eat it.

Whilst many so-called diets are restrictive in terms of social life, e.g. you may struggle to go out for a meal with friends because you're worried about overeating, intermittent fasting doesn't come with that problem attached. You can go out, provided you schedule it for your eating window, and you can eat what you want, within reason. Obviously, you can't go around eating three pizzas simply because there are no rules, but a couple of slices is fine!

There are many different types of intermittent fasting, and the only major difference between them is when you can eat. There are no rules in terms of what you can eat; these types all allow you to eat at different times, or different quantities of time. For instance, some might advocate a full day of fasting, perhaps twice per week, whilst others will simply ask you to fast for x number of hours every day. In this case, you need to pick the type which suits your lifestyle best. We're going to give you the low down on what that means. For now, you simply need to know that this is probably the easiest intermittent fasting method around, and it's also arguably the most popular as a result.

Chapter 1:
Different Types of Intermittent Fasting

Lean-Gains Method

This intermittent fasting method focuses on a healthy diet, fasting and rigorous exercises. It is popular because of its ability to convert fats straight to muscle. The main objective of this method is to fast 14-16 hours every day from when you wake up.

Waking up and fasting up to 1 pm and doing a warmup and stretches just before midday is a perfect approach to this method. From midday, do any exercise of choice for up to one hour and break your fast at 1 pm.

From there, go about your day's activities normally, and when it is around 4pm, eat again. Eat again at around 9 pm. This will give you about 15hours of fast until 1 pm on the following day. If it is challenging at the beginning, you can start fasting for 13 hours for several days and then increasing to 15 hours.

14:10 Method

In this method, you fast for 14 hours and eat during the other 100 hours. It works in a similar way as the 16:8. The difference is that the eating period in this method is 10 hours as opposed to 8 hours in 14:8.

20:4 Method

Whereas 14:10 method was an easier step down from 16:8 method, 20:4 method is absolutely an increase in terms of difficulty. It's a more intense method certainly, for it requires 20 hours of fasting within each day with only a 4-hour eating window for the individual to gain all his or her nutrients and energy.

The majority of the people who opt to use this method end up having either one large meal with several snacks or they have two smaller meals with fewer snacks. 20:4 is flexible in that sense—the sense whereby the individual chooses how the eating window is divided amongst meals and snacks.

20:4 method is tricky, for many people instinctually over-eat during the eating window, but that's neither necessary nor is it healthy. People that choose 20:4 method should try to keep meal portions around the same size that they would normally have been without fasting. Experimenting on how many snacks are needed will be helpful as well with this method.

Many people end up working up to 20:4 from other methods, based on what their bodies can handle and what they're ready to attempt. Few start with 20:4, so if it's not working for you right away, please don't be too hard on yourself! Step it back to 16:8 and then see how soon you can get back to where you'd like to be.

The Warrior Method

The warrior method is quite similar to 20:4 method in that the individual fasts for 20 hours within each day and breaks fast for a 4-hour eating window. The difference is in the outlook and mindset of the practitioner, however. Essentially, the thought process behind the warrior method is that, in ancient times, the hunter coming home from stalking prey or the warrior coming home from battle would really only get one meal each day. One meal would have to provide sustenance for the rest of the day, recuperative energy from the ordeal, and sustainable energy for the future.

Therefore, practitioners of warrior method are encouraged to have one large meal when they breakfast, and that meal should be jam-packed with fats, proteins, and carbs for the rest of the day (and for the days ahead). Just like with 20:4 method, however, it can sometimes be too intense for practitioners, and it's very easy to scale this one back in forcefulness by making up a method like 18:6 or 17:7. If it's not working, don't force it to work past two weeks, but do try to make it through a week to see if it's your stubbornness or if it's just a mismatch with the method.

12:12 Method

12:12 method is a little easier, along with the lines of 14:10, rather than 16:8 or 20:4. Beginners to Intermittent Fasting would do well to try this one right off the bat. Some people get 12 hours of sleep each night and can easily wake up from the fasting period, ready to engage with the eating window. Many people use this method in their lives without even knowing it.

To go about 12:12 method in your life, however, you'll want to be as purposeful about it as you can be. Make sure to be strict about your 12-hour cut-offs. Make sure it's working and feeling good in your body, and then you're invited to take things up a notch and try, say, 14:10 or maybe your own invention, like 15:11. As always, start with what works and then move up (or down) to what feels right (and even possibly better).

5:2 Method

5:2 method is popular among those who want to take things up a notch generally. Instead of fasting and eating within each day, these individuals take up a practice of fasting two whole days out of the week. The other 5 days are free to eat, exercise, or diet as desired, but those other two days (which can be consecutive or scattered throughout the week) must be strictly fasting days.

For those fasting days, it's not as if the individual can't eat anything altogether, however. In actuality, one is allowed to consume no more than 500 calories each day for this Intermittent Fasting method. I suppose these fasting days would be better referred to as "restricted-intake" days, for that is a more accurate description.

5:2 method is extremely rewarding, but it is also one of the more difficult ones to attempt. If that works better for you, don't be ashamed to embrace it! However, if you're dedicated to having days "on" and days "off" with fasting and eating, there are other alternatives, too.

Eat-Stop-Eat (24-Hour) Method

The eat-stop-eat or 24-hour method is another option for people who want to have days "on" and "off" between fasting and eating. It's a little less intense than the 5:2 method, and it's much more flexible for the person, depending on what he or she needs. For instance, if you need a literal 24-hour fast each week and that's it, you can do that. Meanwhile, if you want a more flexible 5:2 method-type thing to happen, you can work with what you want and create a method surrounding those desires and goals.

The most successful approaches to the eat-stop-eat method have involved more strict dieting (or at the very least, cautious and healthy eating) during the 5 or 6 days when the individual engages in the week's free-eating window. For the individual to truly see success with weight loss, there will have to be some caloric restriction (or high nutrition focus) those 5 or 6 days, too, so that the body will have a version of consistency in health and nutrition content.

On the one or two days each week the individual decides to fast, there can still be highly-restricted caloric intake. As with the 5:2 method, he or she can consume no more than 500 calories worth of food and drink during these fasting days so that the body can maintain energy flow and more.

If the individual engages in exercise, those workout days should absolutely be reserved for the 5 or 6 free-eating days. The same goes for the 5:2 method. Try not to exercise (at least not excessively) on those days that are chosen for fasting. Your body will not appreciate the added stress when you're taking in so few calories. As always, you can choose to move up from eat-stop-eat to another method if this works easily and you're interested in something more. Furthermore, you can start with a strict 24-hour method and then move up to a more flexible eat-stop-eat approach! Do what feels right, and never be afraid to troubleshoot one method for the sake of choosing another.

Alternate-Day Method

The alternate-day method is similar to eat-stop-eat and 5:2 methods because it focuses on individual days "on" and "off" for fasting and eating. The difference for this method, in particular, is that it ends up being at least 2 days a week fasting, and sometimes, it can be as many as 4.

Some people follow very strict approaches to alternate-day method and literally fast every other day, only consuming 500 calories or less on those days designated for fasting. Some people, on the other hand, are much more flexible, and they tend to go for two days eating, one day fasting, two days eating, one day fasting, etc. The alternate-day method is even more flexible than eat-stop-eat in that sense, for it allows the individual to choose how he or she alternates between eating and fasting, based on what works for the body and mind the best.

This more intense style of fasting works particularly well for people who are working on equally intense fitness regimens, surprisingly. People who are eating more calories a day than 2000 (which is true for a lot of bodybuilders and fitness buffs) will have more to gain from the alternate-day method, for you only have to cut back your eating on fasting days to about 25% of your standard caloric intake. Therefore, those fasting days can still provide solid nutritional support for fitness experts while helping them sculpt their bodies and maintain a new level of health.

Spontaneous Skipping Method

Alternate-day method and eat-stop-eat method are certainly flexible in their approaches to when the individual fasts and when he or she eats. However, none of those mentioned above plans are quite as flexible as spontaneous skipping method. Spontaneous skipping method literally only requires that the individual skip meals within each day, whenever desired (and when it's sensed that the body can handle it).

Many people with more sensitive digestive systems or who practice more intense fitness regimens will start their experiences with IF through spontaneous skipping method before moving on to something more intensive. People who have very haphazard daily schedules or people who are around food a lot but forget to eat will benefit from this method, for it works well with chaotic schedules and unplanned energies.

Despite that chaotic and unorganized potential, spontaneous skipping method can also be more structured and organized, depending on what you make of it! For instance, someone desiring more structure can choose which meal each day they'd like to skip. Let's say he chooses to skip breakfast each day. Then, his spontaneous skipping method will be structured around making sure to skip breakfast (a.k.a.—not to eat until at least 12 pm) daily. Whatever you need to do to make this method work, try it! This method is made for experimentation and adventurousness.

Crescendo Method

The method is very well-suited for female practitioners (since their anatomies can be so detrimentally sensitive to high-intensity fasts). Essentially, this approach is made for internal awareness, gentle introductions, and gradual additions, depending on what works and what doesn't. It's a very active, trial-and-error type of method.

Through crescendo method, the individual starts by only fasting 2 or 3 days a week, and on those fast days, it wouldn't be a very intense fast at all. In fact, it wouldn't even be so strict that the individual would have to consume no more than 500 calories, like with 5:2, eat-stop-eat, and others. Instead, these "fasting" days would be trial periods for methods like 12:12, 14:10, 16:8, or 20:4. The remaining 4 or 5 days out of the week would be open eating-window periods, but again, the practitioner is encouraged to maintain a healthy diet throughout the week.

Crescendo method works extremely well for female practitioners because it enables them to see how methods like 14:10 or 12:12 will affect their bodies without tying them to the method hook, line, and sinker. It allows them to see what each method does to their hormone levels, their menstruation tendencies, and their mood swings. Therefore, the crescendo method encourages these people to be more in touch with their bodies before moving too quickly into something that could do serious anatomical and hormonal damage.

Crescendo method will work extremely well for overweight or diabetic practitioners, too, for it will allow them to have these same "trial period" moments with all the methods before choosing what feels and works best, based on each individual situation.

Chapter 2:
Introducing The 16:8 Method

If you do any research into intermittent fasting methods, and there are quite a few, you'll find that the 16:8 method comes up first on most lists. You might also see this written as Lean Gains, but it is one and the same thing.

The 16:8 method is an intermittent fasting type, and it comprises of a cycle of fasting and eating normally. When following the 16:8 method you are not told that you cannot eat certain foods, and you're not told that you should eat specific foods either. The choice is yours and that means you have the freedom to change up your eating habits according to what suits you. Of course, this does not mean that you can go around eating all the unhealthy foods simply because the diet doesn't specify! Moderation is something you need to exercise at all times, and something which will become far easier as you start to notice weight loss.

Weight loss is a cumulative effect in so many ways. When you see changes in your body and you see the scales start to change, you'll want to keep up the good work and momentum. That means you're far less likely to 'fall off the wagon' and opt for something unhealthy, and you will start to feel far better for kicking out the unhealthy foods too. You'll notice that your body feels better when you eat healthy fruits and vegetables when you choose whole grains over white bread, white rice, etc, and you'll feel far less sluggish for not eating chocolate, crisps, and carb-laden foods. Of course, you can treat yourself occasionally, but the chances are you won't want to!

You see, healthy lifestyles actually become quite addictive!

What is The 16:8 Method?

Now it's time to get into the real nitty-gritty of what this method actually entails.

We've mentioned that there are many different types of intermittent fasting, and some do actually ask you to fast for 24 hours, a few times a week. The 16:8 method differs because there are no long and arduous fasts, you simply fast for 16 hours every day, and eat normally for 8 hours.

Now, that sounds a lot, 16 hours, but you are going to be sleeping for most of it! You see, you can move the fasting period to suit your needs. We'll talk about how to follow the method in more detail shortly, but a good example is someone who needs to eat breakfast versus someone who doesn't specifically want to eat early in the mornings. We're all different, but most of us fall into one of these two categories. You might wake up starving hungry and need breakfast otherwise you can't focus, or you might wake up and simply need a coffee, and you feel a little sick if you eat straight away.

There are two ways you can manage this, just to give you an example of what the 16:8 method looks like.

If you need breakfast, you can eat it as soon as you wake up, kickstarting your 8-hour eating period. So, if you wake up at 8 am, you have breakfast at 8.30am, and that means you need to finish eating by 4.30pm. You might go to bed at 10 pm, which means you're only consciously fasting 5.5 hours. As you can see, it's not as horrendous as it sounds, and you can drink water, non-calorie containing drinks, and unsweetened, black tea or coffee during your fasting times too. It's actually highly recommended that you drink plenty of water anyway because dehydration is not something you want to play Russian roulette with!

The other scenario is that you are someone who doesn't really want to eat when they wake up. In that case, you can get up, get dressed, have a black, unsweetened coffee, and you can skip breakfast, starting your eating window at lunchtime. So, for instance, you would begin eating at 12 pm. This means you can eat freely until 8 pm. You would then perhaps sleep at 10 pm, which means you're effectively not consciously fasting too much!

This is why the 16:8 method is so popular.

Of course, during your 8-hour eating window, you need to be mindful of what you're eating. If you cram those 8 hours full of crisps and chocolate, then you're going to eat far more calories than you should in the full 24 hours of the day, and you're probably going to gain weight, rather than lose it! If however, you're mindful of what you eat, not particularly being restrictive, but simply thinking more along the lines of health, you'll be full and satisfied by the end of your eating window and read for your fast. This means you will lose weight quite easily and grab the overall benefits of intermittent fasting too.

Why is This Method Best For Beginners

The 16:8 method is one of the easiest to follow and easiest to understand, which is why many beginners choose it. Of course, it doesn't suit everyone and because one size doesn't fit all, it might be that some people switch to a different method after a short amount of time. That's fine, and that might be something you want to think about. so always bear in mind that if you find the 16:8 method isn't working as well as you want it to, for you, then there are other alternatives.

For the most part, however, the 16:8 method, or Lean Gains, is very successful for many, and it is a method which encourages healthy eating without rules and regulations in terms of restriction. There are no massive changes to lifestyle, which is something which many people struggle with when they try a different eating routine, e.g. the Keto Diet, Atkins, Paleo, etc. These all come with a lot of rules and regulations and there are lists of what you can and can't eat, and how it should be prepared. This can overwhelm many a beginner and cause them to rebel against it and say: 'no thanks!' The 16:8 method and many other intermittent fasting methods don't come with those rules attached. There is no weighing or counting required, simply making healthy decisions, which aren't rocketing science. For example:

- Pizza is bad, brown bread is better
- Chocolate is bad, the fruit is better

- Cakes are bad, vegetables are good

Can you see how easy it is? It's not rocket science to make healthy choices, and that doesn't mean you have to be 100% healthy all the time! Want a burger? Have one, but only once a week, and make sure the rest of that day is packed with healthy foods.

The other plus point is that the 16:8 method doesn't have to bother your social life. Most people want to head out with friends or their partner for dinner on occasion, or perhaps out for a few drinks, but this can be very difficult when following a low calorie or fad diet. With the 16:8 method, all you need to do is ensure that you schedule the get-together for your eating window. This might be more difficult if you're starting your eating window early and finishing early, but you can always meet up for lunch instead of dinner! There aren't restrictions on what you can eat, but in most restaurants, you can always make healthy choices on the regular menu.

Let's sum up the main reasons why most beginners opt for the 16:8 method.

- It's easy to follow and doesn't require any counting, weighing, or monitoring
- You can alter your eating time according to your needs
- You can set much of your fasting period into your sleeping period, so you don't notice it quite so much
- The eating method doesn't need to interfere with your social life too much at all
- You are not restricted on what you can eat, provided you make sensible, generally healthy choices

- It doesn't feel like a diet, it feels more like a new lifestyle with timings, rather than food you can and can't eat
- You can still have calorie-free drinks, water, and unsweetened, black tea or coffee
- You won't notice hunger quite so much with this type of eating plan, as there are no extremely long fasts involved

Chapter 3:
How to Follow The 16:8 Method

The 16:8 method is very flexible, and that means you can choose your own specific 8-hour eating window, according to your day. You might work shifts, and that means you sleep at different times. What you should do in that case is pick an 8-hour window which is when you are mostly awake. Obviously!

For example, if you are working nights and you are sleeping between the hours of 10 am and 6 pm, that means you can eat from 6 pm until 2 am. You would then probably be working until the following morning when you would head off to sleep, but you could drink coffee (unsweetened and black) to keep you going also, and plenty of water. You could then choose an eating window of 9 pm and eat freely until 5 am.

It's really up to you!

We've already covered the two main methods most people try with the 16:8, and that is the skipping breakfast and starting to eat at lunchtime routine, or in the case of someone who really needs breakfast because they can't concentrate without it.

It's not only about when you can eat, but it's also about what you eat too. Whilst there are no restrictions and no lists of foods you must eat and foods you shouldn't, always remember that if you suddenly pile a huge breakfast or lunch on your plate after fasting, you're going to end up with stomach ache. That could mean that you end up eating too many calories within your eating window and actually put weight on, or you end up with stomach disturbances for the rest of your eating window, don't get enough fuel during that time because your stomach is so bloated you can't bear to eat. It's about choosing carefully, which we'll talk about a little more shortly.

So, how many calories should you eat? It depends on whether you want to lose weight or maintain. A standard calorie amount to maintain weight is 2500 calories per day for a man and 2000 calories per day for a woman. This does depend on the height, current weight, and metabolism of the person, and is really only an average, healthy amount. If you want more solid guidelines on your specific circumstances, speak to your doctor, who will be able to give you a calorie aim plan tailored to your needs.

Within that calorie amount, you should make sure that you get a good, varied diet. That means proteins, carbs, fats, vitamins, and minerals. Again, we're going to cover what you can and can't eat, loosely because there are no rules, shortly, but varied is the way to go. Ironically this will also help you enjoy your new lifestyle more, because you're not bored and eating the same things all the time. This is a pitfall many people suffer from regular low-calorie diets; the change is so restrictive that they end up eating the same thing day in, day out, and over time they get so bored and simply rebel against it. This usually ends in a binge day which causes extreme guilt and then leads them to throw the diet in the bin and go back to eating whatever they want.

Whilst following the 16:8 method you should also make sure that you drink plenty of water throughout the day, whether fasting or eating.

This ensures that you don't become dehydrated and will also aid in digestion. In addition, you should also exercise too!

Now, there are no rules to say that you must exercise whilst following an intermittent fasting routine, but it will help you lose weight faster, and it will help with your general health and wellbeing. Exercise is fantastic on so many levels, not least helping to build lean muscle, which also boosts your ability to burn fat as an energy source. Exercise is also known to help with mental health issues, such as anxiety and depression, as well as stress. We all live stressful lives, and a little exercise can sometimes be enough to reduce it to levels which are extremely manageable. Aside from anything else, exercise can be a sociable and fun activity!

So, let's sum up how to follow the 16:8 method quickly.

- Eat for 8 hours per day, consecutively - you cannot break these hours up, they must be observed as one block of time
- Fast for 16 hours per day, again, this needs to be done consecutively
- You can choose when you take your 8-hour eating block, but it's a good idea to stick to the same times every day, so your body gets into a routine
- Your fasting times should coincide with sleeping, to cut down on the amount of conscious fasting
- Do not be afraid to miss breakfast, in this eating routine, there is no 'important meal of the day', there is simply an important eating window

- You can drink unsweetened, black tea and coffee, water, and other non-calorie containing drinks freely throughout your eating and fasting times, and you should certainly consume enough water throughout the day to ensure you don't become dehydrated

- During your eating period, you should spread your meals out carefully, so you don't 'binge' when you initially break your fast. This will only lead to stomach aches and other unpleasant gastric symptoms!

- Choose healthy meals as much as possible, but there are no restrictions on what you can eat. If you go unhealthy, however, remember that you're not going to create the calorie deficit required for weight loss

- Whilst you don't need to count calories whilst following the 16:8 method, it's worth bearing the standard calorie amounts in mind, which is 2500 for a man and 2000 for a woman, every day, as an average

- You should also exercise if you want to gain extra health benefits and speed up weight loss also

- Never be tempted to cut down your eating window or to restrict your calorie amount beneath the average - this will lead you towards extreme hunger and also borderline starvation is you refuse to eat. Remember, fasting is not starving!

Autophagy and fasting

Autophagy

Autophagy is a natural physiological process involving the cleaning up in the body of aged or damaged substances. Although it sounds a little unnerving, the literal translation of autophagy is' self-eating.' It is derived from the Greek words auto, which translates to' self' and phagein, which means 'eating.' The term autophagy was coined by Christian de Duve, a Nobel Prize-winning scientist after a group of researchers noticed an increase in lysosomes (parts of the cells responsible for breaking down excess or worn out organelles, food particles, and engulfed viruses or bacteria). Autophagy plays a crucial role in preserving the body's homeostasis — a healthy and stable internal environment. Your body constantly has proteins and organelles (small, complex structures in each cell in your body) that become defective or die. If these dead tissues are allowed to accumulate in the body, they can cause cell death, contribute to poor tissue and/or organ function, and even become cancerous. During autophagy, the body identifies damaged parts of the cells and unused proteins in the body. Such broken sections are sent to lysosomes, where they are cleaned out of the body. This procedure prevents them from causing harm.

Dr. Colin Champ, Certified Radiation Oncologist and Assistant Professor at the University of Pittsburgh Medical Center, describes this process as an innate recycling program. He believes that the autophagy cycle makes your body more effective by eliminating any defective parts, preventing any metabolic disease (such as obesity and diabetes) and avoiding ageing (and possibly cancer) There is also proof that autophagy can play a role in decreasing chronic inflammation and improving natural immunity. Research shows that subjects who are unable to induce autophagia to tend to carry more weight, sleep frequently, and have higher levels of cholesterol and reduced brain function.

Chapter 4:
Tips and tools to stay focused

The most important thing you can do to guarantee your progress in intermittent fasting is to have a plan in place.

The very first step is to decide what kind of fasting you're going to do. Once you have decided on the method of fasting, create a timetable. Do you want to fast every day? What times are you going to fast and what times are you going to feed?

After you've established a timetable, another critical component is to decide what you're going to eat when it's time to enter your fed state. Are you planning to follow a strict dietary regimen (such as a low carb diet or a Paleo Diet) or are you going to stick to a simple diet plan with no real' rules?'

Incorporating food planning

Once you've got the basics down, planning your meals will help keep you on track and discourage you from looking for unhealthy food in periods of hunger. Research shows that people who plan their meals in advance experience greater progress in their health and nutrition objectives and also save time and money in the end. As you get into the rhythm of intermittent fasting and your new way of life, you will make adjustments to your diet and your schedule.

Tips for preparing meals

Organizing the dinner is one of the most important components of good meal preparation. It might seem overwhelming, or like a waste of time, to sit down and arrange ingredients and type everything out, but it'll end up saving you time on the road.

The amount of food you buy in preparation and the amount of time you spend preparing is entirely up to you. Many people spend three to four hours on Sunday preparing meals for the whole week.

Irrespective of what kind of meal you choose, organization is the key.

Find out of your strategy

First, you'll have to structure your supper plan. You can design out a couple of days, seven days, or then again even for the whole month. Discover basic plans and record all that you'll be eating and at what time. At the point when you're first beginning with intermittent fasting and feast arranging, the energy may entice you to search for extravagant, new plans or a great deal of assortment, yet when you're in the underlying phases of another way of lifestyle change, one of the most advantageous things you can do is adhering to the fundamentals and not over complicate things. Stick to foods that you're as of now acquainted with and plans that won't take as well long to get ready or that expect you to adapt new kitchen abilities or purchase new kitchen equipment. There's a lot of time for you to attempt new things after you become accustomed to the rudiments and your body and brain conform to the changes. The purpose of supper preparation is to make you feel less overwhelmed, not include any unnecessary pressure. There are online meal planners and trackers just as mobile applications that you can use to monitor your suppers, however, you needn't bother with any fancy apparatuses or software if technology isn't your thing. You can keep it straightforward by recording everything in notepad.

Write Your Grocery List

When you've gotten your plans together and your feast plan worked out, it's time to make sense of what you need. Check your refrigerator and your pantry before composing your staple rundown so you don't buy things you already have. After you've arranged a rundown of things you have close by, work out a staple rundown of the remaining things you'll have to finish your plans and your meals for the week (or then again for whatever time allotment you've picked). You can spare much additional time by sorting out your basic food item list depending on where things are found in the store. You can list all meats together, all produce things together, and every single refrigerated thing together. In case you have to go to various stores for any arrangements or any special grocery, sort out your list at the store.

Prepare your meals

A great way to save money is to shop the same day you'll be preparing your meals. This way, when you get home, you won't have to put away as many food items— you can jump right into preparing your meals. After the meals have been prepared, split them by portion size into separate containers and appropriately mark them. So when you're ready to eat, you'll have breakfast ready to go and it'll be easy to transport if you're bringing lunch with you on the go.

Take photos and measurements

If weight reduction is one of your objectives, don't depend entirely on the scale. Your real weight can vary fundamentally from every day, and you probably won't see enormous changes in the numbers in any event, when your body is experiencing a massive change. You can utilize the scale as an instrument, yet take these everyday numbers while taking other factors into consideration. Rather, take "before" and "after" (or "progress") pictures. Pictures can be truly motivating tools since when you see yourself consistently, you may not see the little changes happening, however, when you analyze pictures that were taken a month, the progressions might be fundamentally increasingly obvious. Try not to let any present disappointment with your body prevent you from taking before pictures. You'll be glad you have them not far off. Notwithstanding pictures, it's useful to take body measurement.

You may begin to achieve a slender size, particularly if you're working out or engaging in strength training normally. As your body begins to transform, you may not see an over the top move on the scale, yet your body composition can change significantly. Measurement can assist you with the following advancement in achieving inches loss from various regions of your body. You'll need to take the following measurement:

- Bust: measure right around your bust, keeping the estimating tape in line with your nipples.

- Chest: measure exactly underneath your breast or pectoral muscles and the entire path around your back.
- Waist: discover the tightest piece of your waist, normally directly beneath your rib cage, furthermore, measure right around.
- Hips: locate the vastest region of your hips and measure right around.
- Thighs: measure right around the fullest piece of your upper leg while standing upright.
- Knees: measure right around straightforward over the knee while standing straight.
- Upper arms: measure right around the fullest part of your upper arms over your elbows.
- Lower arms: measure right around the fullest part of your lower arms

Underneath your elbows. To appropriately measure, you'll need an unstretchable measuring tape. Keep the tape level around your body and parallel to the floor. At the point when you're taking your measurement, fold the tape over your body as near your skin as could reasonably be expected, be that as it may, don't crush so firmly that the measuring tape cuts into your skin or makes a space. It's useful to have another person take your estimations for you so you can stand straight; in the event that you don't have somebody accessible, take your measurement before a mirror to ensure that you're keeping the tape level and estimating in the right spots. Make a list of your estimations in a journal or on your mobile phone's note pad. Take your estimations at regular intervals and record the numbers in a similar place without fail. As time goes by, you can utilize the measurements to help visualize your progress.

Expect some disappointments

Like anything in life, with intermittent fasting, you can encounter ups and downs, particularly at the very beginning. Don't assume all to move right off the bat perfectly and don't get lost in perfection. You'll slip up: sometimes you'll snack outside your feeding slot, and that's all right.

If you go into it, realizing you're trying to put your best foot forward but still recognizing it may take a while to get used to the change, you're going to be less likely to beat yourself when things don't go absolutely according to schedule.

Chapter 5:
First 30 Days Of Intermittent Fasting Program Schedule

Week 1

In the first week, you'll only conform to the window

Tasks

1. Choose your favorite eating window for eight hours. Note that your fasting time is dedicated to sleep. Try to base the feeding period on moments where you know it's going to be difficult not to feed and exercise.

2. Don't dramatically change the type of food you eat. It's about getting used to the food window this week.

3. Do not attempt exercise if you are new to the practice of fasting, the most probable surge in appetite may find restraint more challenging. Only focus on sitting in your room.

4. Practice Monday–Friday's 16:8 approach and have the weekend off

Week 2

If you were able to stick to the tasks outlined in week 1, then continue to the tasks listed below. We're going to address sleep this week and start the 16:8 food pattern.

Tasks

1. Assess the feeding period for the last weeks. You've got to change it? Is it in accordance with your schedule? If so, start Monday-Friday to use this opportunity. If no, select a new period for feeding and replicate week 1.

2. Implement one of the four suggestions outlined earlier in this Monday–Friday.

3. If you have itchy feet, feel free to exercise gently! Nonetheless, if you are dealing with a hunger to enable your feeding period to be fully adapted, I would still suggest no workout.

4. Also, don't radically change the type of food you eat.

Week 3

We're going to add exercise this week. You probably hanged out to blow some calories if you haven't begun already

Tasks

1. Open the nutritional slot. Does this still work? Must it alter to make you become more disciplined? Start with your current window Monday-Friday if the window is perfect. If not, choose a new window and go back to week 1.

2. Depending on your ability level, incorporate sufficient HIIT instruction, build a two-three-fold exercise this week.

Remember; please check with a qualified doctor before implementing every food or exercise plan. For your visit to the FREE HIIT program:

3. Start to cut back on sugar. This task varies from person to person.

Week 4

You should have the ideal eating period in position by week four. If you are still suffering, I strongly suggest that you get a group's assistance in week 3.

Task

1. Continue eating the time you have selected Monday-Friday

2. Add some of the foods listed for adding magnesium and potassium

3. Under electrolytes. Find choices for balanced dessert to help you stay happy! Here, the trick is to find keto desserts because they are high in fat and weak in carbohydrates. Keep in mind the fat spikes less insulin and makes the body turn to energy storage. Don't buy the policy of "low fat."

4. Implement a second tip outlined for better sleep. (My favorite person is more sunlight).

5. Continue to remove sugar

6. Conduct 2-4 HIIT exercises

The first 30 days of 16:8, as you can see, are not drastic. I didn't describe giving up pasta, potatoes or even sweet treats. In order to keep you inspired to start, you will invest your first 30 days making improvements and getting great results. How to get going is the key to long-term success. While I know how hungry you are for success, I caution against pushing forward as a novice. First of all, the number one reason people give up is seeking too much, too fast. Sometimes, we've been overweight or unhealthy for 5-20 years. In the blink of an eye, it is unrealistic to expect long life patterns and lack of discipline to be changed.

Chapter 6:
Benefits of Intermittent Fasting

What is the point of intermittent fasting? Well, that's easy. The primary reason that people start to take an interest in intermittent fasting is for rapid weight loss. And why not? Many individuals, both male and female, do struggle with maintaining healthy weights.

Is that the only reason to try intermittent fasting? Absolutely not! Intermittent fasting can provide the body with several benefits. Some of these benefits are felt and seen in day to day life, like weight loss, losing belly fat, and reduction of inflammation. Yet, there are benefits that work on a more long term scale.

Studies have shown that following an intermittent fasting cycle reduce blood sugar levels, reducing the risk of blood sugar related complications. Additional studies have shown that intermittent fasting has the potential to reduce the risk of Alzheimer's disease.

So, intermittent fasting can help with both short term and long term health! The results can be rapidly noticeable, as well.

Increased Weight Loss

Okay, so you've tried diets for weight loss before. What makes Intermittent Fasting different from all the other diets that have come and gone? Well, first of all, Intermittent Fasting isn't a diet; it is a lifestyle! Get that notion of 'diet' of the brain. A lot of people hear or read the word 'diet,' and they immediately discredit the information.

Now that we have moved past the concept of 'diet' and are sticking to the idea of a lifestyle, what makes the 16/8 Intermittent Fasting plan ideal for weight loss?

Well, 16/8 refers to the fact that in 24-hour days, 16 hours of the day are spent fasting and 8 hours are allotted for meals and snacks. That may not seem like much, but between full-time work schedules, getting the kids to and from school, visiting friends and family, eight hours can fly right by!

Generally, a popular time cycle for the 16/8 intermittent fasting lifestyle is scheduling the fasting time to include the 8 or so hours you spend sleeping.

So, the non-fasting eight hours is most popularly scheduled during the workday. It can be difficult to eat more than one large meal during a work shift. Therefore, while following this popular schedule, most people will skip a morning meal, have a large afternoon meal with some snacks before and after and then forgo a large evening meal or have a smaller evening meal.

One large meal and some snacks throughout an 8 hour period will tend to consist of far fewer calories and carbohydrates than eating three big meals and additional snacks. That in itself is a start to the weight loss process and one of the reasons the 16/8 intermittent fasting plan can be so effective.

What happens when we consume food? Well, digestion is a rather complex process, but the part that is relevant to an intermittent fasting cycle is how carbohydrates from food are transformed into glucose.

Glucose feeds the cells of our bodies, giving them the energy to carry out their designed function.

While cells do need glucose to power themselves, they aren't high-performance machines. A car can only drive so many miles on a gallon of gas. The rest of the gas in the tank just hangs around until it can be used. Cells can only burn through so much glucose at a time.

When eating bigger meals and snacks, the body has the potential to take in far more carbohydrates than the cells can process. Unlike a car gas tank, the cells don't just hold onto the glucose until it can be used. Excess glucose gets turned into fat stores in the body, contributing to weight gain and belly fat accumulation.

Without restricting eating times or allowing for fasting cycles, the body cells are likely to default to the fresh, new glucose being provided every time a meal or snack is consumed. Whatever glucose has become a fat store is just going to sit there unnoticed, accumulating more fat.

Looking back at intermittent fasting, when the body isn't taking in more carbohydrates to become glucose, the cells don't stop functioning. Cells continue to work and do their jobs, but they still need fuel. So they turn to other fuel sources. These sources are the accumulated fat stores.

So why is the 16/8 intermittent fasting cycle ideal? Well, the body can take up to 10 hours to start processing its fat stores. Fasting for 16 hours gives the body ample time to start processing fat stores and burn through a portion of them.

Great, so we know how fasting contributes to weight loss and how restricting the eating time contributes to weight loss. Well, how do they work together? Why is the 16/8 intermittent fasting plan better than the other options out there?

The theory is, when the body fasts for 16 hours, it is able to burn through fat stores. Then when food is consumed for 8 hours in smaller portions and with fewer calories and carbohydrates, the fat stores don't build up at the same rate they are being burned. As you can see, this method if fasting ensures that the fasting cycle and non-fasting cycle both contribute to weight loss.

Looking at some of the other plans, if you fast for 2 days a week, during those 48 fasting hours, plenty of fat can be burned, but nothing restricts you from replenishing those fat stores the other 5 days during the week.

As you can see, a continuous cycle of intermittent fasting, like the 16/8 cycle can ensure maximum weight loss because it approaches the issue from two angles.

Now consider the Keto Diet. Ketogenic diets are based on the concept of the body only consuming about 20 Carbohydrates a day. This is stricter than just following an intermittent fasting cycle; however, it can really supercharge weight loss!

Carbohydrates provide the cells with Glucose. The keto diet can kick weight loss up a notch because, during the 8 hours of non-fasting, fewer carbohydrates mean less fat going into storage. It also means that by the time you enter your fasting cycle, the cells might already be looking for more fuel, so it could take less than 10 hours for them to start burning through fat stores.

The 16/8 Intermittent Fasting plan provides a multi-faceted approach to weight loss and fat burning, encouraging greater success. The weight loss process can be expedited by following a low carb diet alongside your fasting cycle.

Increased Longevity

The idea of living longer is popular in many societies. Pharmaceutical companies develop medications to reduce aging side effects. Cosmetic companies created lotions and creams to reduce and reverse wrinkles. Hair salons work with a lot of clients who color their hair regularly to hide grey and white as aging changes hair color. To more extreme levels, plastic surgeons provide services such as Botox and body modifications that provide a younger, firmer appearance.

People want to live longer.

However, after all, said and done, plastic surgery, medications, and cosmetics don't really stop the body from aging. Bodies do age, and no one has come up with a cure for an age yet.

That doesn't mean increasing personal longevity and lifespan are fantasies that are out of reach. In fact, intermittent fasting has been known to aid in increased longevity! How strange is that? Actually, it isn't as odd as it sounds.

Intermittent Fasting and restricted eating plans do have something in common. Whether you are intentionally counting calories or just carefully following your 16/8 intermittent fasting plan, calories do tend to get restricted when eating and fasting this way.

Good news! Caloric restriction has reportedly been the most efficient way to combat aging!

How does Calorie Restriction combat aging? Well, the aging process is about as complex as the human body itself. That is to say; it is very complex. Aging isn't fully understood in the scientific community, just like the human body. There is always more to learn, but what we do know now is that restricting calories impact five mechanisms that contribute to human aging. Caloric restriction supports these five mechanisms in a way that promotes much healthier and longer aging cycles.

The five mechanisms that caloric restricting impacts are:

- Cell Proliferation
- Mitochondrial Physiology
- Inflammation
- Antioxidants
- Autophagy

I know, those sound pretty heavy in terms of scientific terminology. Fortunately, all five of these mechanisms are interrelated with each other and in human aging.

Cell proliferation is also referred to as Growth Balance. When cells are in an anabolic state, they are powered up for building organs and tissues. Cells remain in an anabolic state when there is an abundant supply of calories, like when we eat regular meals and snacks.

With regular fasting and caloric restriction, cells are allowed to enter their catabolic state. Cells in a catabolic state are breaking down, recycling, and repurposing tissues.

Allowing the body proper cycles to break down and repurpose old tissues and then cycle into building up new tissues perpetuates a healthy cycle of regenerating tissues, thus provided longer life to organs and body tissues.

Mitochondria are parts of cells. They are organelles that are needed to create ATP or cellular energy. This ATP allows the cells to work and powers cells in both physical and cognitive labor.

As the body ages, it starts to impair mitochondrial network quality. When the network quality diminishes, the breakdown of damaged and dysfunctional mitochondria is decreased as is the body's ability to build new mitochondria.

Intermittent fasting and caloric restriction help both the destruction and creation of damaged and new mitochondria, respectively.

Animal studies have shown that since cells are exposed to less glucose during fasting, the ATP production does drop off for a while. This triggers a process in the cell to replenish ATP and allow cells and mitochondria to better produce ATP in the future. Kind of like a computer reboot but of the ATP production in a cell.

As the body ages, joints and other body parts begin to experience damage from use and wear and tear over the years. To protect the body, the immune system begins to create inflammation. In itself, inflammation is not bad as it is a natural protective response the body has to injuries.

Unfortunately, as the body ages, damage and injury accumulate and become more prevalent. In an attempt to protect itself, the immune system keeps producing inflammation, sometimes contributing to chronic inflammatory diseases.

Fasting and calorie restriction has an inhibiting effect on one of the nuclear factors that exert anti-inflammatory effect. Basically, reducing this nuclear factor's (Nf-kB) activity through calorie restriction forces the signals in the immune system that create inflammation under-regulated, producing less inflammation. Less inflammation means the aging body is less prone to chronic inflammatory issues.

Intermittent fasting and calorie restriction help antioxidant defenses. During the aging process, reactive oxygen species increase and antioxidant defenses decrease. As this imbalance grows, damage accumulates (creating inflammation) and mitochondria begin to malfunction faster (mitochondrial physiology).

Trying to balance the reactive oxygen species with antioxidant defenses helps with mitochondria function and preventing chronic inflammation. That's where intermittent fasting and calorie restriction comes into play again! Calorie restriction promotes antioxidant defenses by activating nuclear factor (Nrf2), which regulates the cell's ability to resist oxidants.

In regards to autophagy, which translated at its root words quite literally means 'self-eating. As autophagy progresses, old cell structures and cell junk are removed. This junk can accumulate over time and hinder cells from performing at their highest level. This is where fasting and growth hormone become beneficial.

During a fasting cycle, the human growth hormone is amplified and kind of on overdrive. When this hormone kicks on, it signals the body to produce replacement parts for the pieces that are being scrapped during autophagy. This includes mitochondria.

Autophagy is basically a recycling process for the cellular structures in the body. Since it relies heavily on growth hormone to actually recycle and repurpose the old, junky parts, then having growth hormone in an amplified state is beneficial to the process.

Here you can really see how these different mechanisms are interrelated. Thus, using intermittent fasting to restrict calories has a widespread benefit over the aging process and contributes to longevity.

Human Growth Hormone Production

Human growth hormone was touched on as being an important part of cell growth and regeneration through autophagy. The human growth hormone is vastly important to the body in other ways than just keeping the cells replenished and functioning smoothly.

The human growth hormone is produced in the pituitary gland in the brain. Levels of human growth hormone are higher in the body when children are growing. These levels peak during puberty, when the body goes through its most drastic hormonal changes. After puberty, the human growth hormone begins to dwindle in the body. This is normal in adults, but that doesn't mean the hormone isn't still beneficial.

The human growth hormone is suppressed during non-fasting periods because its function is to increase the blood glucose level. When calories and carbohydrates are being consumed, the human growth hormone goes on standby.

Fasting periods stimulate the secretion of the human growth hormone. This hormone is beneficial as it has a positive influence on the muscles, encouraging them to recover quickly. This specific benefit is important to anyone who is an athlete or exercises regularly.

Additionally, adults who are human growth hormone deficient tend to have higher levels of body fat and lower levels of lean body mass as well as less bone mass.

While all hormones are released periodically in the body naturally as a mechanism to prevent the body from building up a resistance, it is possible to have hormone deficiencies. That is why intermittent fasting can be beneficial in raising the growth hormone levels.

In as little as 5 days of fasting, the human growth hormone can have an increase of 300%. That is a lot in a short amount of time, so even in just 16 hours of fasting, human growth hormone production will go up.

The human growth hormone helps in anti-aging, or healthy aging. It also helps the muscles recover for people who are athletes or regularly active. In one 6-month study of the human growth hormone in people, the group receiving hormone injections and the control group didn't exhibit differences in weight. However, the differences in lean mass vs. fat mass were quite noticeable.

Those receiving the human growth hormone injections increased their lean mass (muscle mass) by about 8.8 percent more than the control group. Their fat mass had an average 14.2% decrease and a loss of 5.3 lbs. of fat mass! The skin even exhibited thickening.

So, there it is, the human growth hormone can and does contribute to a reduction in fat mass and an increase in lean mass. This is great for anti-aging, but also anyone looking to decrease their body fat levels and increase their muscle mass. Of course, working out and exercising while intermittently fasting will also enhance muscle mass, especially with additional production of the human growth hormone.

Fasting is the best way to naturally stimulate the production of the human growth hormone. This hormone is crucial to child development, puberty, and continued functionality in the body into adulthood.

It doesn't take extensive fasting periods for the human growth hormone to start being produced. Therefore, sticking to the 16/8 intermittent fasting cycle will include the human growth hormone benefits.

Chapter 7:
How Weight Loss Is Achieved in General?

Before we look at the best way that you can use intermittent fasting to help you reduce your body fat percentage, let's first quickly consider how weight loss generally works – think of this as the science behind effective and guaranteed weight loss.

When you eat something – regardless of what it is – it means you are putting calories into your body. Nutrients are broken down and absorbed by your body, while carbohydrates are broken down and then processed into glucose, which is then distributed through your body to provide cells with energy.

When excess glucose is present in your body, it will usually be stored as fat cells through a rather complicated process that we are not going to be discussing in detail here. As fat cells increase, you gain weight – ultimately leading to you becoming overweight and then slowly obese.

Now, on the other hand, when you are physically active – whether you are walking, dancing, or going hard on the treadmill at the gym – you are burning calories. Your body uses more glucose for energy, and when the reserves run out, the body starts looking toward stored fat cells in order to generate more energy. This energy then allows you to continue running on that treadmill or allows you to pick up the set of weights a few more times.

So, to sum this up – you eat, you gain calories; you exercise, you lose calories.

When the number of calories you eat surpasses the number of calories you lose, then you gain weight. Think of this within a 24-hour cycle. If you eat 2,000 calories, but only burn 1,000, then you gain weight to the value of those extra 1,000 calories that are left behind at the end of the day.

When you eat more calories than you burn, it means there is a caloric surplus. You are gaining weight and cannot lose weight with this strategy.

To lose weight, this entire equation needs to be in an opposite manner. You need to lose more calories than you burn. If you eat food that calculates to around 2,000 calories each day, you need to burn more than the 2,000 calories if you wish ever to see your fat go away and the number of the scale go down.

When your daily calorie intake is less than the number of calories you lose, then it means you have a caloric deficit – this is the ideal goal that you are striving toward when you are aiming to reduce your body weight.

Intermittent Fasting and Weight Loss Through a Caloric Deficit

You should have a basic understanding of how weight loss works – that you need to create a caloric deficit if you ever wish to see your weight go down.

Now, let's take a quick look at how intermittent fasting plays a role in this entire process. With intermittent fasting, you still need to create a caloric deficit. I've seen some people think that simply because they are fasting, they will lose weight, regardless of the other factors in their life. This is not true.

No matter how beneficial fasting might be and a program that utilizes intermittent fasting, you will still need to take the science behind weight loss into account. If your caloric intake is more than how many calories you lose in a day, then you set the way for weight gain and not weight loss.

Intermittent fasting can make things a little easier, however. It has been found that people who follow an intermittent fasting program eventually experience improvements in their level of satiety. Their appetite is reduced, in other words. Since weight gain often lies within the fact that a person is unable to control their urges to eat inappropriate times, the reduced appetite will certainly be beneficial.

Additionally, because all meals of the day need to be squeezed into an eight-hour window with the particular intermittent fasting method that I am focusing on in this guide, it usually means that you will still feel somewhat full with your second meal after you had your first. When the time comes to have your third meal, the second meal will still be satisfying your appetite a little. You'll end up not wanting to overload your plate every chance you get – this means it becomes much, much easier than before to be in control of how many calories you will be consuming on a day-to-day basis.

Strategies for losing weight quickly

Some strategies make your life easier by reaching your target of weight loss quickly. It's important to look healthy and happy with a thinner body. These strategies are to be noted and memorized on your fingertips. The two main strategies that have a huge contribution to weight loss are increasing your fasting window and having a high-calorie deficit. All the other tips will be summarized along with the main points.

Increasing your fasting window will definitely lead to weight loss, but not with the powerful biological effects of intermittent fasting.

At the initial stage, start your fast after dinner so that it passes as you sleep and also improves your adherence to dieting. Keep your window short to around 12 hours, especially if you are a woman.

Stick to a routine by setting up one. Start and break your fast at regular timings every day. The routine will also keep you away from boredom. It's tough to manage time when you have work, family life, and other life circumstances, but here we have the benefit.

One way is to slowly increase your fasting window to 16 hours. The other way is to keep changing the timings every day according to routine.

The third way is to fast for the number of hours you desire every day, following your hectic working hours, starting from 12 hours onwards. This way you can adapt to many routines and set the plan for your entire week. Set day one with a fasting period of 14 hours, day two with 12 hours, day three with 18 hours and so on.

When you have the will, you can find the way and get that chic body you have to give in your best. If you cannot handle it, get yourself a dose of caffeine early morning and in the afternoon.

The 16/8 method is famous for being similar to the normal routine with no difficult challenges as such.

HELENA is to date, the most extensive research done on Intermittent Fasting. The German Cancer Hospital was also involved in the process but is not in favor of the diet routine in the long run. 150 obese individuals were examined for the study and divided accordingly into three groups. The first group followed a calorie restriction method that reduced the calorie intake by about 20% through the 16/8 protocol. The second group was supposed to follow the 5:2 plan or alternate fasting routine. The third group being the control group just had to take a balanced diet.

The purpose of the study was to find out whether intermittent fasting is a healthy way of reducing weight. The results turned out to be surprising.

Both the methods proved to be equal in terms of health and weight loss effects. The belly fat reduced too. Some people may find it easy to control themselves within 2 days only instead of a whole week adjustment. It is better to switch to a balanced diet anyhow. Kuhn, the leading scientist of the research thinks that it is best to choose a dietary method and keep consistency. He says that the health effects will be achieved any way from the weight loss so why not choose something that benefits the lifestyle.

Having a high-calorie deficit will directly lead you to weight loss. Weight loss by the loss of the excess body fat is completely healthy and also releases greater energy during its breakdown. This keeps the dopamine, a neurotransmitter, satisfied as it is responsible for the control of emotions. It's critical to have micro and macronutrients added to your diet, but a high-calorie diet will spoil it all. Although you have the leverage of eating bread, rice, pizza, pasta, etc. it is always beneficial and effective to approach the protein-rich diet. These high carbohydrates food items not only raise your blood sugar, blood pressure, and fat, but also cause extreme mood swings and depression. This does not mean you cannot have any carbohydrates or fat. It just reminds you to have healthier options. For intermittent fasting, this can be beef, fish, fruits, veggies, avocados, and almonds. Nuts are healthy fats that provide a lot of calories with just a small portion, and therefore their intake should be kept in minimal quantities. Soups are a convenient option for a meal replacement as they provide lesser calories than solid foods and are satiating too.

Other power tips include keeping yourself hydrated enough to lower your appetite and for the body to perform its functions. The water intake gives your stomach the perception of being full, which signals the brain regarding the feeling. Green tea can also make the experience way easier than it is by suppressing and curbing your hunger pangs. The overall process shall increase your body's metabolic efficiency. During your fed state, it is tough to manage fat burning as your insulin levels are increasing, so the only duration that gives you a chance for fat burning is your fasting state. After your last meal, the body enters the post-absorptive state where the body has a low insulin level and is not ready to further process any more meals. Having more meals and snacks will raise insulin levels and instead of breaking down, it will be stored as fats. Eat carefully as your body will always prefer burning sugars before any other source.

Therefore, no carbohydrates should be eaten. Without any readily available glucose or glycogen units, your body will have no choice, but to force the fat cells to breakdown for energy. Post-workout, the glucose in your muscles has already been depleted as the aerobic and anaerobic respiration used it, but the meal we will be consuming now will either be stored to replace the burned glycogen in the muscles or will be broken straight away. Therefore, post-workout meals even if they are high in calories are always good to have.

Let's just switch to lettuce and broccoli as our favorites rather than Margherita pizzas with pepperoni. Thus, the conclusion of the strategies is that when you do eat, it should be with mindfulness and moderation while overdoing nothing (including fat). Get your 8 hours of sleep and feel rested. Do not over exhaust yourself.

After having gone through 40 studies review by Harvard Chan School of Health, it was found that intermittent fasting was an efficient measure for weight loss. Individuals would lose within 7lbs to 11lbs over 2.5 months. They have also figured out how the locking of the mitochondria in one state can block the effects of intermittent fasting.

Chapter 8:
Nutrition and dietary recommendations

Protein recommendations:

A common mistake when trying to lose weight is to overeat protein. As mentioned earlier, excess protein can be converted to glucose (sugar) and stored as glycogen. Due to the difference in atomic composition, glucose cannot be converted into proteins. Use the equations below to calculate your protein needs based on your goal. Weight loss = 0.36 g to 0.70 g per pound of bodyweight PURPOSE. Example: Mandy weighs 198 pounds, but has a target weight of 174 pounds. 0.36 x 174 = 62.64; 0.70 x 174 = 121.8 The ideal daily intake of Mandy's protein is 62 - 122 g. Mandy must now have at least 62 grams of protein per day to maintain muscle, but no more than 122 grams per day to prevent the conversion of protein into glucose. Bulk weight = 1.5 g to 2 g per pound of bodyweight PURPOSE. Example: John weighs 165 pounds, but has a target weight of 200 pounds.

Carbohydrate recommendations:

The calculation of carbohydrates can be complicated because it varies from person to person. Below are some guidelines that you can follow. Keto = 30 g or less per day. They must come primarily from green leaves. This method is a principle from a ketogenic diet. Plateau Destroyer = 100 g or less per day. This should mainly come from green leaves and resistant starches. This principle is useful when you have reached a plateau. Beginner = remove refined sugars. Rather than focusing on macros, a starting approach should be to eliminate refined sugar and take up resistant starches.

Eat saturated fat:

Fully hydrogenated fats become saturated fats. They do not contain trans fats. If it remains stable at average room temperature, it can be considered as saturated fat.

Examples of healthy fats:

- Avocado
- Fatty fish
- Olive oil
- Coconut oil
- Thick yoghurt
- Nuts
- Whole eggs
- Cheese

Cooking guide:

Saturated fat is the safest cooking ingredient. Unlike other fats and oils, fats do not saturate when exposed to heat.

Fruit Tips:

The simple fact is that fruit contains a lot of sugar. At the molecular level, your cells do not divide foods, such as fruit and chocolate, into ' healthy' and 'unhealthy' categories. Glucose is glucose, period. Any other form of sugar, fructose, dextrose and any other word ending with "bone" is converted to glucose and used accordingly. Fruit should only be consumed in season and tiny quantities if you are trying to lose weight. Our bodies are involved in the use of fruit as a loading medium in the cold months when there is not enough food. Our body is unaware that we live in a society where we have access to food all year round. And constantly eat fruit, talk to your body, that should move in a state store because the winter is coming. Here's how I recommend you use fruit when it comes to fruit smoothies to lose weight. Zanja consumes direct fruit after training with a protein shake. Never eat fruit without a protein source. Fruit smoothies are sugar bombs. The amount of sugar cancels out any antioxidant effect that the drink can have. Use green leaves to get the same benefits. Eating fruit after training with a protein shake is a great way to increase insulin so that muscle cells can absorb a protein shake. I know that the increase of insulin, as a rule, the red light, when fasting, to lose weight, but in this case, will help to increase muscle mass, because insulin also is responsible for assisting cells in absorbing proteins. If you want to eat fruit as a snack, make sure you eat it with a protein source, such as nuts. This reduces the absorption of sugars into the bloodstream, gives it longer energy and prevents the loss of energy at the end of the day.

Calorie Goal Formula

If you wish to get more technical and have some time on your hands to do a rather simple calculation, then I suggest you follow a specific formula in order to calculate a more accurate daily calorie goal. This will essentially be more useful than using generic advice.

You will then adjust the BMR according to your activity level, and then make another adjustment for the goal you are trying to achieve – which is to lose excess fat, in this case.

To do this, you'll have to determine your lean body mass and your fat percentage. To calculate your lean body mass, follow this formula: current weight – (current weight x (your current body fat percentage / 100). You'll then calculate your BMR with this formula: 370 + 21.6 x LBM (your Lean Body Mass that you calculated in the previous step.

Once you have your BMR, consider how active you are. If you are sedentary most of the time, then the formula is your BMR times 1.2. For light activity, BMR times 1.375. For moderate activity, BMR times 1.55. If you are very active, then BMR times 1.725.

All you need to do now is take your body fat percentage into account. If your body fat percentage is higher than 30%, then lower the number of calories calculated in the previous step by 30%. If you are between 20 and 30%, then lower calorie intake by 25%. For 10 to 20%, lower by 20%, and for those with a body fat percentage that is under 10%, lower your calorie intake by 15%.

The result is the number of calories you should ideally eat every day in order to ensure you can lose weight.

Sound too complicated? Let's take a look at a quick example.

Let's call our sample person Joey. Joey weighs 120kg and has a body fat percentage of 32%. Joey only participates in light activities throughout the week.

Lean Body Mass: 120 – (120 x (32/100)) = 81.6

BMR: 370 + 21.6 x LBM = 2132

Activity adjustment: 2132 x 1.375 = 2931

Daily Calorie Recommendation: 2931 – 30% = 2052

Determine What Foods You Should Include In Your Meal Plan

Now that you have set up the appropriate calorie plan for yourself, it is time to move forward. You will now have to start setting up a food plan for yourself. let's first take a look at some of the most ideal foods that you should try to have in the meal plan you are planning to follow.

I just want to provide you with a few foods that are known to accelerate fat loss. These are the types of food that you should try to include in your diet in order to promote an improvement in your metabolism and to essentially help to speed up your weight loss results.

Instead, they will form somewhat of a basis or an outline for preparing meals. You'll still enjoy other types of food (not the fattening kind, however), and then add some of these foods to your meals to promote improvements in your efforts to lose weight.

Leafy Greens

Of course leafy green deserves its place at the top. Leafy greens include a range of different vegetables like collards, spinach, swiss chard, and kale. These are, without a doubt, some of the healthiest foods that you can eat, and they are excellent for anyone who is trying to shed some excess pounds.

The thing with leafy greens is these vegetables are very low in calories. They are also not loaded with carbohydrates like some vegetables and fruits are. On the other hand, leafy greens contain a lot of fiber, which is not only good for your digestive system but can also be an extremely useful tool in helping you shed those extra pounds that you had packed.

One scientific paper looked at numerous studies that have been conducted in the past and confirms that there is a positive relation between fiber intake and body weight. With a higher fiber intake, obesity can be prevented more effectively. Among people who are obese, an increase in fiber intake may yield a positive interaction with their body weight – both body fat and body weight tend to decrease among obese individuals who start to follow a high-fiber diet.

The paper explains that the primary mechanism in terms of how fiber assists in weight management lie with the ability of the substance to reduce appetite. When food intake is decreased through a higher fiber consumption, there are less excess calories in the body to be stored as fat at the end of the day.

Cruciferous Vegetables

Another class of vegetables that should definitely be included in your meal plan if you intend to lose weight would be cruciferous vegetables. These generally include Brussels sprouts, cabbage, broccoli, and cauliflower. All of these vegetables are also very good for your entire body and may yield positive results in terms of your weight loss efforts.

Cruciferous vegetables are, similar to leafy greens, loaded with high-quality plant-based fiber. This means that including more of these vegetables in your meal plan will help you feel fuller after you have had a meal. The end result is a decrease in your daily caloric intake.

In addition to being a great source of plant-based fibers, cruciferous vegetables can also help you increase your intake of protein, another important nutrient that is definitely crucial for any type of weight loss program.

A paper published in the American Journal of Clinical Nutrition explains that a diet that contains relatively high amounts of protein can be very effective in aiding a person in their weight loss program, and can also be an effective mechanism for weight management in general.

The study explains that protein intake should be equal to around 1.2 to 1.6 grams of protein per one kilogram of body weight, with an approximate minimum protein per meal suggested to be around 25 grams. In turn, this amount of protein can assist in various elements that are related to weight management, including:

· Appetite will be reduced and, in turn, lead to a lowering of the daily caloric intake

· Risk factors associated with cardio-metabolic health are improved

· Body fat can be reduced when combined with an appropriate meal plan and, of course, a physical activity program

A Boiled Potato

Potatoes are often thought to be "bad food" when it comes to weight loss, but when used the right way, a simple boiled potato can actually help you reach your weight loss goals. The important thing to do here is to boil the potato and then allow it to cool for some time before you consume it.

When a boiled potato cools down, it leads to the formation of a type of substance known as resistant starch. This is similar to fiber and will be able to improve your satiety – that said, you'll feel full for some time, allowing you to get through your day without opting for foods that will simply add to your calories and cause weight gain.

A potato will give you vitamin C, calcium, iron, and there are two grams of fiber in a medium-sized potato – this is excluding the resistant starch that will be formed when you allow a boiled potato to cool down.

The phytonutrients found in potato will further benefit you, and there are antioxidants that can help to fight against free radicals in your body, promoting heart and brain health, while also fighting against cancer and many other diseases.

Intermittent fasting reduces the development and progression of tumors in animal experiments. Rats on IF transplanted with a cancer cell line survived longer than free-fed animals. After 10 days, 50% of the IF animals were still alive compared to 12.5% in the control group.

Alternating fasting used only in middle age mice reduced the incidence of lymphoma in mice. In a 4 month observation period, 30% of the control mice became ill while none of the animals on intermittent fasting became cancerous. The researchers also found a better antioxidant activity, resulting in less development of harmful free radicals within the mitochondria (cell power plants). The antitumor effect did not result from the calorie reduction since both groups consumed the same amount of calories.

In rats, intermittent fasting reduced the development of pre-neoplastic (precursor to cancer) liver injury and liver nodules caused by a carcinogenic substance.

Unfortunately, human studies have not been conducted so far.

In one study, intermittent fasting in non-obese participants resulted in an increase in good HDL cholesterol in women and a reduction in triglyceride levels in men. This effect occurred over 22 days for every two days fasted. This change may have been caused by the degradation of body fat, which was -4%.

In the case of obese people, the values improved more clearly by an average weight loss of -5.6 kg after eight weeks of alternating fasting.

Total cholesterol dropped by 21%, LDL cholesterol by 25% and triglycerides by 32% while HDL cholesterol remained unchanged.

The systolic blood pressure dropped from 124 to 116 mmHg.

Stress resistance induced by intermittent fasting has a cardio protective effect beyond reducing body weight. Studies in mice show that in a heart attack, the affected tissue in the heart is half-smaller in alternately fasting mice than in normally fed animals. Also, in cardiac infarction, 4 times fewer cardiocytes die (heart muscle cells), when the animals were fed intermittently.

Meal Planning

Meal planning, also known as meal prep, is NOT required to be successful with intermittent fasting, however, it does a good job of preparing you for even more success with your feeding window. Meal prep is preparing some or all meals/snacks in advance to have on hand when needed. Meal prep saves you time, so you aren't preparing meals/snacks each day and it takes away the thought process of what you will eat during your feeding windows daily. By meal prepping, there is less room for failure, especially for beginners. With meal planning comes the bonus of preparing healthier options to eat during your feeding window, instead of choosing quickly processed and prepacked options because it's convenient.

For me there are many steps to Meal Planning. Meal Planning consists of creating full meals (this includes recipes), creating all-inclusive grocery lists, reviewing your own kitchen to see what you already have and what you need, then altering your grocery list, and finally going grocery shopping.

Creating meals takes creativity. With the world wide web, there are plenty of recipes and meals ideas for available options. Being creative means not always eating the same thing day in and day out. Change up your breakfast options, lunch options, dinner options, and snacks.

Season the food differently. Cook a different cut of the beef. Garnish it differently. Make it a soup or salad instead of a casserole. Make vegetables a snack in some way. Find ways to increase your protein intake. Add more green leaves to your protein shakes and/or more vegetables or fruits. Decide on 2-3 lunch and dinner options, and 2-3 snack options.

Once you have decided on what meals you have created and the recipes, you will need to search through your kitchen cabinets, freezer, pantry, and refrigerator to see what you have already have and don't need to purchase when you go food shopping. This includes everything, meats, sides, fresh vegetables, fresh fruit, drinks, snack options, spices, herbs, oils, breads, wraps, and more. Revise your grocery shopping list to include what you need.

Proceed to go to the grocery stores and pick up the items on your list. In preparation for meal prep. Meal prep is taking all of your groceries and cutting up everything that needs to be cut up, washing everything that needs to be washed, marinating everything that needs to be marinated, seasoning everything that needs to be seasoned, baking everything that needs to be baked, cooking everything that needs to be cooked, measure everything that needs to be measured to the appropriate portion, and packing it all in individual meal Tupperware containers to easily grab and go when needed. Although highly recommended, meal planning and prep, is NOT required for intermittent fasting.

Choose Food Options Wisely/Balanced Options

When following an intermittent fasting lifestyle, you are not restricted from any food group and you can choose your own meal options, BUT food choices are still (as always) important. It is important to have good nutrition that emphasizes a diet that provides a complete source of minerals, vitamins, and nutrients for the healthiest functioning body.

A diet is considered the sum of all foods eaten, but it refers to the use of specific intake of nutrition. Any healthy diet should include whole and unprocessed foods over processed and/or liquid foods to include plenty of fruits and vegetables, lean proteins, some fats and oils, and grains; this would be considered a balanced meal, these are also called energy-dense foods. Energy-dense foods are high in fiber and helps to retain natural water.

When fasting, try to eat more non-starchy vegetables and lean proteins. Choose foods that are whole grain and stay away from refined grains and flours. Fruit is going to be the best option to try to curb the still existing sweet tooth, especially for beginners. Choose a non-dairy over dairy and eat fats and oils in moderation and choose the healthiest forms of fats and oils.

Fresh fruits and vegetables are favored over frozen and canned, but any vegetable is better than no vegetables at all. Choose lean cuts of protein and to increase your protein intake add vegetarian sources, like beans and soy products. Try almond, soy, or cashew non-dairy options to limit your dairy intake, as dairy is one of the world's leading allergens. Other leading allergens include eggs, peanuts, and shellfish. Make carbs toppers instead of the base of your meals. When buying pasta, bread, crackers, and more, always look for whole grain listed as the first ingredient on the nutrition label. Eat half of an avocado at least once a day to increase your healthy fat intake.

Chapter 9:
Common Mistakes to Avoid When Fasting

Many people who are just starting their fasting cycle, tend to make beginners mistake, which can result in goals not being achieved and many other hosts of things. If you are beginning with intermittent fasting, chances are you will make those mistakes. Meaning, for it to not happen, it is best that we talk about it and show you ways to combat it. With that being said, let's talk about the first mistake.

Start intermittent fasting quickly

Many beginners make the mistake of starting intermittent fasting way too fast, and when they begin to quickly, it becomes unsustainable for them to continue with intermittent fasting. If you have started anything immediately, you might have noticed that it became tough for you to follow, which led to you not continuing. Same goes for intermittent fasting, and you need to make sure you take the right steps before you jump into following intermittent fasting. With that being said, let's talk about many ways beginner intermittent fasters tend to start too quickly. The first mistake they make is by picking a fasting protocol, which is way out of their Realm.

As we talked about before, you need to ease into intermittent fasting, especially if you're women. You cannot expect to fast for 24 hours when you have never even fasted in your life, so start small. It is always recommended that women begin with 12-hour fast, or if that sounds too intense for you can start to by meal skipping. You have to make sure that, whatever you follow it is done gradually, so you don't quit. Another way people tend to start intermittent fasting too quickly is by not Consulting the doctor. Believe it or not, their chances that you might not be healthy enough to follow intermittent fasting.

That is why it is advised that you consult a doctor before starting fasting; for example, if you have diabetes, you are not advised to begin intermittent fasting. There are many health complications which not allow you to follow intermittent fasting, that is why we always recommend you ask a doctor before you start intermittent fasting or it can be very devastating.

Beginners also tend to extend the fasting window very quickly; if you haven't fasted for more than four weeks comfortably, then it is not recommended to extend the fasting window. We need to take into consideration that for beginners, going from 12 hours to 16 hours can be a drastic difference. That is why it is always advised that you stick with a fasting protocol for an extended period, ideally for four weeks. If you make the jump of increasing hours too soon, you will notice it becomes tough for you to continue with fasting and you might give up.

Overeat during the eating window or too little

People make the mistake of eating a lot or too little when following intermittent fasting, and the truth is it is straightforward to do either. People who are looking to lose weight will eat less during their eating window, thinking that it will help you lose more body fat. Whereas overeating will not make up for all the fasting, you did throughout the day. Which is why it is imperative that you do none, so in this section, we will teach you how to make sure you aren't doing either when following an intermittent fasting protocol.

Now, even though fasting allows you to eat whatever you want when you break your fast, it still essential to make sure you eat correctly. You see if you try and eat junk food and try and hit your macros, it would be tough for you not to overeat. Let me explain how that works, as there is something called a high glycemic carb which most of the junk foods. What these high glycemic carbs are responsible for is digesting very quickly in your body, which spikes the insulin very fast.

When you absorb and shuttle the foods to quickly as you would with junk food, you will get hungry very fast, which would make you overeat. Which is why it is best advised that you eat foods which have a lower glycemic index like most healthy meals tend to have. Another thing these healthy foods will help you with would be the fiber, making you feel fuller through the day. Now that we know how not to overeat, let's talk about how to make sure that you aren't under-eating. The first way to make sure that you aren't under-eating would be by counting macros, and this will help you make sure that you are hitting all your calories for the day. Counting macros will ensure you don't under-eat and you don't overeat, it goes hand in hand.

Now, this is the only way to avoid under-eating let's talk about some of the signs you might be experiencing if you under-eat when fasting. The first sign you might notice is that you feel very weak when working out if you follow a workout plan you will see that your strength has gone down which is a tail-tail sign that you are under-eating. Another way to tell that you are under-eating is if you know that you feel less energy throughout the day, rather than feeling more heat. One of the many benefits of intermittent fasting is the fact that you can get a lot more power, but it won't work if you are under-eating. So by now, you can tell that overeating and under-eating aren't optimal for fasting. Which is why you need to make sure that you stay on track with your macros when fasting, the other tips we gave you work great as well.

But do whatever works for you to ensure that you aren't under eating or overeating, and there are millions of way to go about it. Find an eating routine which helps you feel full, and allows you to eat just the right amount of calories to where you are getting closer to your goals instead of drifting away from them if your goal is weight loss or muscle gains you need to make sure your calories are the right amount. Don't make this beginners mistake as you will regret it, and now you have the tools to ensure you don't make these mistakes

Ignore what for when

One mistake that many people following intermittent fasting make is to ignore what for when. For you to be successful with intermittent fasting, you need to make sure you don't overlook what for when. What do I mean by what for when is simple, ignoring what to do and what not to do when intermittent fasting. We will talk about things to avoid and the things not to avoid when intermittent fasting. More specifically, we will teach you how to listen to your body.

You are ignoring what for when is merely a metaphor, nonetheless an important one. First of all, when intermittent fasting doesn't jump too quickly from fasts to fasts. Most beginners make the mistake of not riding out the protocol for a substantial amount of time before they jump to conclusions. Make sure that you have done at least four weeks of following this protocol as it will show you how your body reacts to this fasting method.

Before you jump the guns of upping the fasting difficultly, make sure you know how your body works. You need to remember that your body is more important than your goals, so whatever you do, you need to be aware of what your body is telling you. Don't do anything which makes you feel like you are harming your body, and as always consult with your physician before you start a fast.

The first way to not mess up on overeating would be to make sure that you are counting your macros. This is one of the best ways to make sure you stay on track with your eating habits during your fasting windows. When you have calculated your macros and following them accordingly, you will have a lot better chance of not under eating or overeating during your eating window. Another way to make sure that you are not overeating is to eat slowly, and many people tend to get extremely excited when they see food in front of them during their eating window. It is best advised that you don't indulge in them and more than you should.

Not drinking enough water

Drinking water is crucial when your intermittent fasting, is there a lot of benefits to drinking water. It also helps you care about your appetite. We will talk about the reasons why you should be drinking more water when intermittent fasting, and also show you why you might not be drinking enough water and techniques to allow you to drink more water when fasting. Many people know that water is very beneficial to humans, water help to detox your body clean out your system and also helps you curb appetite. It is crucial that you're drinking more water when fasting. Believe it or not, most of the time you're drinking a lot less water than you required to be drinking. One of the best rules of thumb to follow when you are drinking water is too drink 1 oz per pound of body weight. So if you weigh 150 lbs., you should be drinking 150 ounces of water, especially when you're intermittent fasting; as water will help you forget about food.

Many people know that when you're fasting, especially in the beginning you tend to crave a lot of food. What water will do is help you curb that appetite, so you don't break you're fast prematurely, another thing water will do detoxify your body. When your fasting you're already detoxing a lot of things, if you add more water to it, it will help you detox your body even further making it a lot healthier environment for you. Water will also increase your brain power and productivity, as you know intermittent fasting has shown to improve mental focus so once you add more water to your daily routine, you will notice more focused throughout the day.

Chapter 10:
Why Intermittent Fasting for Women Need to be Different than for Men

Men and women are different. There are subtle differences that are not only physical but emotional and mental between the two genders. Therefore, measuring them both with the same yardstick can become problematic.

The biggest thing that makes the treatment of women differently than men imperative is their ability to bear offsprings. This requires a special body and hormonal structuring and makes all the difference. Therefore, you can talk about all the equality, feminism and all those things, but nothing should undermine the fact that women have a different physical and hormonal structure that needs special attention.

Women have been entrusted with the responsibility to bear kids. The whole process of bearing kids, making it, and providing the required nutrition is heavily fat dependent. A woman's body gets prepared to bear a child as soon as it hits puberty. The body doesn't understand the legal restraints, and it always tries to remain in a state of readiness to bear kids. Till you hit menopause, either you want to have kids or not, your body would always try to attract fat so that whenever conception takes place, it is able to bear a healthy child. This need for readiness makes a substantial difference in the feeding needs of men and women.

Physiologically speaking a woman's body has higher body fat percentage than men. While a man may have an ideal essential body fat ratio of 3-5%, the women may have it anywhere between 10-13%. Even in athletes, male body fat ratio lies between 6-13% whereas female body fat ratio can be as high as 14-20%. In average body type men, the body fat ratio should fall between 18-24%. This ratio in women is between 25-31%. The reason for showing these stats is simple. It is important for women to understand that having a little higher body fat ratio is not only normal but natural. This is how their bodies have been designed. All those women, who are obsessed with zero figures or other such dimensions may be putting their natural body cycle at risk. Therefore, whenever a woman thinks of losing weight, this fact should be kept in mind.

Another thing that mandates that women have a different fasting schedule than men is their hormonal system. The hormonal cycle of women is highly sensitive to hunger signals. They are more sensitive to starvation, and their bodies are designed to bear kids, and that cannot be possible when there is a shortage of food. Therefore, longer and difficult fasts would hurt your fertility and childbearing abilities.

This makes it necessary that women always move ahead with fasting schedules very slowly.

They should never start with longer food gaps without practice.

They must always increase their fasting period in small progression.

They should not be adamant about continuing fasting for the complete duration.

Women shouldn't keep fasts longer than 24 hours as that can seriously mess up their hormonal cycle.

If these things are followed, even women can follow intermittent fasting easily.

Effect of Fasting on the Hormonal System of Women

Fasting tells the body it isn't a good time for fertility. When you fast for long, and your body starts having an energy deficit on a consistent level, it starts conserving the energy for necessary functions and fertility is not one among them. This has been proven through several studies that prolonged fasting can lead to shrinking of ovaries.

However, it is important to clarify here that these experiments have only been conducted on mice. The induced fasting time was only of a few days, but on the life scale of mice, it could have meant fasting for much longer.

However, besides everything else, it is an undisputed fact that fasting for long is a problem for women. There are several hormones that get affected. The estrogen levels get messed up if the fasting is not done carefully or calorie restriction is carried out.

Here, it is again important to clarify that this imbalance can happen with any calorie restriction followed by women. It means regardless of the method followed like diet, calorie restriction or intermittent fasting, such problems can arise if due attention is not paid to the process.

Imbalance in the hormonal levels can have a wide impact. The practitioners may face metabolic disorders, weight loss ability, mood, bone density, energy, cognitive function, anxiety, and stress levels all may get affected.

Impact of starvation on various hormonal balances would be:

Impact of estrogen imbalance

- ✓ Low energy
- ✓ Poor heart health
- ✓ Infertility
- ✓ Poor glucose regulation
- ✓ Weight gain
- ✓ Reduced skin and hair health
- ✓ Poor cognitive function
- ✓ Decreased bone density
- ✓ Poor muscle tone

Imbalance can also trip the Cortisol levels in your body. It is the stress hormone. The impact would be:

- ✓ Sugar cravings
- ✓ Low energy
- ✓ Anxiety
- ✓ Fatigue
- ✓ Insomnia

Thyroid imbalance can also take place. It may lead to:

- ✓ Weight gain

✓ Brain fog

✓ Depression

✓ Anxiety

✓ Dry hair dry skin

✓ Irregular periods

✓ The feeling of cold or hot flashes

Fasting is a very healthy practice. Intermittent fasting is an even improvised version of fasting to eliminate the harmful things so that only beneficial things can be retained. However, incorrect observation of any procedure will lead to negative fallouts. Therefore, it is important that women should follow intermittent fasting in the right way and very carefully. They need to be more observant about the changes and never become lax in their approach.

Fasting tells the body it isn't a good time for fertility. When you fast for long, and your body starts having an energy deficit on a consistent level, it starts conserving the energy for necessary functions and fertility is not one among them. This has been proven through several studies that prolonged fasting can lead to shrinking of ovaries. Although the same impact has been visible even in male subjects. However, it is important to clarify here that these experiments have only been conducted on mice. The induced fasting time was only of a few days, but on the life scale of mice, it could have meant fasting for much longer.

However, besides everything else, it is an undisputed fact that fasting for long is a problem for women. There are several hormones that get affected. The estrogen levels get messed up if the fasting is not done carefully or calorie restriction is carried out.

Here, it is again important to clarify that this imbalance can happen with any kind of calorie restriction followed by women. It means regardless of the method followed like diet, calorie restriction or intermittent fasting, such problems can arise if due attention is not paid to the process.

Imbalance in the hormonal levels can have a wide impact. The practitioners may face metabolic disorders, weight loss ability, mood, bone density, energy, cognitive function, anxiety, and stress levels all may get affected.

Impact of starvation on various hormonal balances would be:

Impact of estrogen imbalance

- ✓ Low energy
- ✓ Poor heart health
- ✓ Infertility
- ✓ Poor glucose regulation
- ✓ Weight gain
- ✓ Reduced skin and hair health
- ✓ Poor cognitive function
- ✓ Decreased bone density
- ✓ Poor muscle tone

Imbalance can also trip the Cortisol levels in your body. It is the stress hormone. The impact would be:

✓ Sugar cravings

✓ Low energy

✓ Anxiety

✓ Fatigue

✓ Insomnia

Thyroid imbalance can also take place. It may lead to:

✓ Weight gain

✓ Brain fog

✓ Depression

✓ Anxiety

✓ Dry hair dry skin

✓ Irregular periods

✓ The feeling of cold or hot flashes

Fasting is a very healthy practice. Intermittent fasting is an even improvised version of fasting to eliminate the harmful things so that only beneficial things can be retained. However, incorrect observation of any procedure will lead to negative fallouts. Therefore, it is important that women should follow intermittent fasting in the right way and very carefully. They need to be more observant about the changes and never become lax in their approach.

Intermittent Fasting for Women Over 50

Clearly, women's bodies and digestion change when they hit menopause. Perhaps the greatest change women over 50 experience is they have slower digestion and they begin to put on weight. Intermittent fasting might be a decent method to turn around and forestall this weight gain, however. Studies have demonstrated this fasting design controls hunger and individuals who follow it consistently don't encounter similar longings that others do. In case you are over 50 and attempting to acclimate to your slower digestion, intermittent fasting can assist you with avoiding eating a lot every day.

At the point when you reach 50, your body additionally begins to build up some constants like elevated cholesterol and hypertension. Intermittent fasting has been reported to diminish both cholesterol and pulse, even without a lot of weight reduction. On the off chance you have begun to see your numbers rising at the doctor's office every year, you might have the option to get them down with fasting, even without losing a lot of weight.

Intermittent fasting may not be an extraordinary thought for every woman. Anybody with a particular health condition or who will, in general, be hypoglycemic ought to consult with a doctor. In any case, this new dietary pattern has explicit advantages for women who naturally store more fat in their bodies and may experience difficulty disposing of these fat stores.

Chapter 11
Setting Your Pace

We have now committed ourselves to an intermittent fasting plan, plotted our schedule, and our family are all on board. As we enter our first few weeks of intermittent fasting, it will become clear that our body is taking time to adjust. As we clear our bodies of the confusion of a constant barrage of unnecessary meals and snacks, we will also find that our minds start to become clearer. As it does, you will become more aware of your body's own natural rhythm and you will be able to understand how to pace your fasting in order to maximize the benefit to you.

One of the elements of your body's natural pace is your metabolism. Your metabolism is the name given to a series of chemical reactions that occur within your body that converts food into the energy your body needs to function. Your metabolism can either be an aid or obstacle in your weight loss goals. When a slow metabolism is referred to with reference to weight gain, it means that the conversion of food to energy is slow and, therefore, there is more time for food to be converted to fat if the energy is not burned through. The good news is that intermittent fasting has been shown to increase the rate of metabolic food conversion, meaning that the metabolic rate you were born with can be altered and does not need to be an obstacle to your goals.

The other aspect of pace which is important to address is the cadence that relates to your fast. This is something that we will develop as we move through our journey, but in order to work with our body's internal pace, we need to be consciously aware of how we are feeling and reacting during our fast.

Incorporating Sleep Hours into Intermittent Fasting

Depending on the protocol you have chosen to follow, you may be able to incorporate your hours of sleep into your fast in order to make things easier for you.

It is no coincidence, after all, that we refer to our first meal of the day as breakfast. When we are sleeping, we are essentially fasting; it is just easier because we are not aware of our fast. While we are asleep, our digestive system is quiet and our body is in repair mode. This is very similar to what we are trying to replicate when we practice intermittent fasting. As we start our intermittent fasting journey, it would, therefore, make things far easier for us if we incorporate our sleep into our fast period. If so, you may be reaping the benefits from this choice already. You must continue to assess this choice, though, and ensure that it is still the best fit for you.

Regular fasting can improve our quality of sleep. When we eat shortly before we plan to go to sleep, our digestive systems are active, trying to digest the food we have just consumed. It, therefore, stands to reason that we would not have the same quality of sleep as we would if we had eaten our last meal well before our bedtime.

Fasting is known to assist in strengthening our internal circadian clock. Our circadian clock or circadian rhythm is a 24-hour cycle within our bodies that runs in the background of our brain and determines when we feel alert and when we feel sleepy. A strong circadian clock will exhibit as a person feeling alert at the same times of the day and drowsy or sleepy at the same times of the day/night. It is also known as your sleep/wake cycle. When this circadian clock becomes impaired or weakened, we experience insomnia and other sleep disorders (What is Circadian Rhythm?, n.d.).

When you regularly fast on a schedule, your body becomes more in tune with its circadian clock. As the clock strengthens, we will have an easier time falling asleep, we will have fewer experiences of waking up during the night, and our overall quality of sleep will improve (Breus, 2019).

It is a good idea to eat your last meal and ensure it is nutritious and filling at least two to three hours before you plan to go to sleep. This will ensure that you do not feel too full and uncomfortable when you are trying to get to sleep, but it will also ensure that you do not feel hungry and find yourself focusing on that rather than on sleeping.

As with all new protocols, it may take a few nights for your body to start settling in to the stronger circadian clock produced by fasting, but when it does happen, you will find that you have additional energy and feel far more refreshed when waking.

An issue many people seem to struggle with is waking up in the middle of the night to eat. Waking up ravenous during the night is usually an indicator that you have consumed too few calories during the day. Remember that even though we are practicing intermittent fasting, we are not starving ourselves. We still need to make sure that we are getting sufficient calories to sate ourselves. There is actually an eating disorder involving the compulsive consumption of food at night, so if you find that you are unable to stop from eating during the night, it may be advisable to see a medical practitioner about your symptoms and determine what your triggers for nighttime eating are.

There is, of course, a difference between getting up to snack on an apple and binging on an entire pizza, three bowls of Fruit Loops, and a chocolate bar. Compulsive eating of any kind is never good and the reason behind it must be found and dealt with.

Hydration While Fasting

So much emphasis is placed on how we control our food intake during intermittent fasting that it can be easy to forget about the liquids which form part of our diet. We draw about 25 percent of the hydration we need from the food we eat, so it can be quite easy to become dehydrated when we are fasting. The symptoms of dehydration can include fatigue, headaches, and a dry mouth. It is, therefore, imperative to keep ourselves well hydrated when we fast to avoid these side effects. It is not enough to drink the same amount of fluids as you would when you are not fasting. You must increase the amount of fluids you take in.

Interestingly, there is a link between carbohydrates and water, which explains why we need to take in more fluid when we fast. As we know, carbohydrates are stored in our body as glycogen. For each gram of glycogen stored, we store about three grams of water with it. So when we fast and burn glycogen, we are burning that stored water with it.

This is one of the reasons that weight is quickly shed when carbohydrates are completely removed from the diet. A lot of the weight that you are losing is water weight. That also explains why it is so easy to put that weight back on if you reintroduce carbohydrates into your diet again (Rosenfield, 2019). This is why fasting and calorie and macronutrient counting are a far more sustainable way to lose weight than simply cutting certain things out of your diet completely.

Many studies have shown that eight glasses or eight ounces each are the usual daily requirement of water for a human being. This is just less than two liters. It cannot be overstressed, though, that each individual's requirement is different and you should keep that in mind (Valtlin, 2002). If you find that you are forcing yourself to consume the eight glass amount, then it could be too much for you. By the same token if you still feel thirsty after consuming eight glasses, then your personal hydration requirement may be higher. Do keep in mind that certain illnesses such as diabetes present with symptoms such as excessive thirst, and if you sweat a lot during exercise, you will need to replenish that fluid as well.

What we drink while we are fasting will depend completely on the calorie intake parameters and weight loss goals you have set for yourself. Clean water is always the most ideal hydration method but flavoring with mint, lemon, or cucumber will not necessarily add to the calorie count. Beverages such as tea and coffee will start adding to your calorie count when you drink them with sugar and milk or cream, so you can have plain coffee and tea during your fast. Sodas and other fizzy drinks should generally be avoided and even fruit juice should be watered down as it can often be very high in sugar. These can only be consumed during your eating window period.

When we hydrate ourselves, we are trying to maintain fluid balance. Fluid balance is the balance between the output and input of fluids in the body in order to allow metabolic processes to operate properly. Approximately 52 percent of body weight in females and 60 percent of body weight in men is made up of fluid (Sheppard, 2011).

There are scientific methods that have been developed to determine how much hydration an individual needs but these methods are not yet 100 percent proven as best practice. It is worth looking at one of the methods for the sake of clarity. One method of calculating the amount of hydration a body needs is called the Weight Method or the Holliday-Segar Method. The formula behind this method relates to how many calories are burned in your resting state and equates that to the amount of water lost during this burning of calories. The Weight Method specifies that for every 100 kilocalories burned at resting rate, you require 3.4 ounces of fluid to maintain your hydration. The idea is to take your weight and apply the following formula: first 22 pounds of your weight takes 3.4 ounces of fluid per pound to maintain hydration, the second 22 pounds of your weight takes 1.7 ounces per pound to maintain and, thereafter, each pound requires an additional 0.75 ounces per pound to maintain. MDCalc.com is a website that assists with various medical calculations. It also has a maintenance fluids calculator that makes accurately calculating your maintenance fluid requirements much easier.

This is quite an involved method but it is one of the simplest methods used by nurses to calculate hydration required during hospitalization (David the Nurse, 2018).

Temptations and Interruptions

Snacking is the biggest dietary problem of the modern age. We now have access to an exorbitant amount of quick, easy food and a huge range of snacks that we have started to consume between our meals. This is one of the reasons that we have seen a huge uptake in the rate of obesity in the last 30 or so years. Certainly, we have had things like potato chips and chocolate bars for a very long time but drive-through food facilities are relatively new as are vending machines and a checkout queue lined with unhealthy snacks. Our modern lives have become one huge trap of convenience and consumerism and it's showing in how healthy (or unhealthy) we are becoming.

In any situation where you are trying to exchange old, unhealthy habits for a new, healthier lifestyle, you are bound to come across things that seem out to test you. When we set up our intermittent fasting schedules, we took into account that there could be interruptions to our schedules that would necessitate flexibility. This is one of the reasons that we suggest only setting up a schedule for two weeks in advance so that you can factor in things that come up such as birthday parties or business dinners.

We also addressed getting your friends, family, and coworkers on board so that you can try and avoid temptation as much as possible. A coworker plopping a fat slice of chocolate cake on your desk because it's her birthday when you are in a fasting period could be a serious temptation. You may have told this coworker that you are practicing intermittent fasting but she may have forgotten or she may not have wanted to offend you by excluding you from the festivities. It is in situations like this that we will need to practice some (or a lot of) self-discipline.

In the beginning of our journey, you wrote down all the reasons why you wanted to start intermittent fasting and you visualized those reasons. These writings are going to be a very valuable tool to you when you face temptations or interruptions in your intermittent fasting journey. It is highly recommended that you carry your journal around with you so that you can refer back to the goals you set and the visualizations you created in the beginning of your journey. It is also advisable to write down the temptations and interruptions to your intermittent fasting journey as they come up. If you were happy with how you responded to the interruptions or temptations, you can record how you did this to cement that reaction in your mind. If you feel that you could have handled the interruption or temptation in a healthier way, you can record in your journal how you handled it and what a better way would be to handle it in future.

As you continue with your intermittent fasting journey, you will probably notice that very similar interruptions and temptations come up on a regular basis and you will find it easier to condition yourself into a healthier response that does not disrupt your fast or make you stray from the goals that you have set for yourself.

It may feel easier to simply try and avoid temptations and interruptions rather than to try and learn to deal with them in a healthy way but this is counterproductive in the long run. Temptations can be avoided for a short period but they will inevitably come up again when you least expect them to or they may simply morph into another form and catch you off-guard. This is why it is far better to face these temptations and interruptions head-on and teach yourself to deal with them in a healthy manner so that you are not simply trying to circumvent them. This is also a highly beneficial self-development tool and you will be conditioning yourself to understand that you can handle temptation and not succumb to it.

If you find yourself tempted by the coworker's chocolate cake, remind yourself that thanks to the protocol you have chosen, you are not refusing yourself the cake, you are simply saying that you cannot have it at that very moment.

Remind yourself that you are in control of what you put into your body. Hunger is simply your body's conditioned response to the lack of food that you would normally have at that time. You are in the process of retraining your body and soon it will understand that it does not require food at that very minute. Being aware of how hunger feels and also how fullness feels is very important. When you begin to eat, focus very strongly on exactly how many bites of food you need to take before those hunger pangs start to subside. You may be surprised at how quickly your body no longer feels as ravenous as it did before you started eating. Keep this in mind when you are feeling hungry and remind yourself that it is only going to take a few mouthfuls of food for you to no longer feel that way, so it is not nearly as serious as it seems.

Keep in mind that you are not punishing or restricting yourself; you are liberating yourself from an overload of unnecessary food and you are promoting a process in your body that will lead to an overall increase in your health and longevity. When you think about hunger, keep in mind that what your body has learned to acknowledge as hunger is not always a true need for food. As you have gone through your life, you have conditioned yourself into a pattern of eating. That conditioning has become so entrenched in your body and mind that your body acknowledges it as a true physiological response to a lack of food. What you are attempting to do with intermittent fasting is change that conditioned eating pattern. Remind yourself of this when you think you are feeling hungry.

Chapter 12:
How the intermittent fasting guide is important for your lifestyle

As we began with, intermittent fasting is not only a weight-loss method but also a way to achieve holistic health. By following intermittent fasting, you can remain healthy and fit too. Obesity is not the cause of the problem. The people who are only focused on losing weight and do not try to treat the problems that cause obesity end up regaining the weight pretty fast. They work hard for months and years, but weight loss is never permanent.

For instance, if a person is suffering from chronic inflammation in the fat cells, then losing weight would always remain a big issue for that person. The reason, the inflammation would never allow the person to feel fully satisfied with the food. There will always be an urge to eat more. The more a person eats, the faster will be the weight gain as calorie intake would increase.

Similarly, if a person is suffering from insulin resistance, losing weight would be difficult. The body of that person would always remain in the fat storage mode and hence resist any fat-burning.

These are just some of the examples that clearly demonstrate the fact that if your overall health is good, it would be hard for your body to gain excess weight. The body loves the balance and would try to maintain it in normal circumstances.

Intermittent fasting is a lifestyle change, and hence you must expect some changes in the way you are leading your life. It is always wise to expect that you will have to make some minor corrections in your day to day activities.

When we talk of lifestyle change, it is important that you consider all the aspects of life, eating is just one of them. You will have to change your eating habits. Of late, it has become as if we are living to eat and not eating to live. Food is a primary necessity of life, but it is not the end goal. Living a healthy life that helps you in achieving meaningful goals should be your aim.

To this end, you will have to make some important changes:

Eating Habits

Eating habits, in general, have changed drastically in the past. The food-producing industry has contributed a lot to it. There have been aggressive marketing campaigns about eating smaller but frequent meals. Even increasing carbs in the diet was also promoted at one time even by the government. Although food choices have gone through several changes, eating frequently has become a habit. The food is spread all around us. You can get hundreds of fast food joints on your way that are selling food items that are tempting and cheap. It may not cost you much time and money to grab a bite on your way. However, this habit of munching all the time is taking us towards the health doom. This habit would have to be changed.

Most people are scared of the thought that they may not be able to eat the things they want. In intermittent fasting, it doesn't work like that.

You will still be free to eat practically everything in a limit so that temptation for food can be avoided. However, you will have to follow some reasonable restraint. The habit of eating 'ad libitum' or whenever you desire will have to be controlled. This is very easy when you make some positive changes in your food choices.

In any case, there will not be severe restraints in your eating windows. There is no reason to worry as you will be free to eat the things you want in this period. The major portion of the fasting window passes in your sleep, and hence the chances of temptation are very few and far between. You can expect an easy ride in this section as long as you are ready to curb your habit of frequent snacking.

Food Choices

Most people feel that they'd never be able to get any success through diets as avoiding certain foods is not possible for them. There is no doubt in the fact that food has a strong impact on the physique. We are what we eat. The kind of food we eat eventually becomes a part of our body. Therefore, if you are eating a lot of trashy food, it can never have a healthy impact on you. However, it is also correct that your body has a very robust system of discarding the bad and keeping the good and hence there is a tolerance limit even for bad foods.

So, you can get in shape even if you are taking some liberties in food. However, this should always remain in a limit, and you should always try to eliminate such things from your food slowly.

Refined sugar, alcohol, fried food, highly processed food items, things made from refined flours are some of the things that have a negative impact on your health. You must always try to avoid these things. If that is not entirely possible, you should at least try to limit your intake of such things as much as possible.

Intermittent fasting is not a routine that limits your life. It means that once in a while you can have cheat days and cheat meals where you can eat these things. You don't have to feel cut-off from your friends and social circle because you can't eat certain things. However, you shouldn't make it a habit or a regular occurrence. Things eating in a responsible manner will not have an adverse impact on your health goals.

Healthy Routine and Exercise

Exercise is very important for a healthy body either you are following intermittent fasting or not. Therefore, it is not a contentious subject. Exercise will accelerate weight loss and will also help you in getting healthier. Moderate exercise is good for the functioning of your heart and improving your immune system. Intense physical activity is important if you want to lose a lot of weight fast. It also helps in muscle building.

Exercise helps your weight loss and health goals. However, while fasting certain things need to be kept in mind. Women shouldn't do high-intensity exercises on the fasting days and must keep a one-day interval to give the body complete rest. Exercising in the fasting state is especially very helpful if you are trying to burn fat as the HGH and adrenaline hormone levels are very high in that state. They not only help in burning the fat considerably faster, but they also increase your stamina and boost muscle growth. Detailed tips on exercise and the ones that are especially helpful will be given in the exercise section.

Therefore, including exercise in your daily routine is always very helpful. The kind of exercise you want to do would depend upon your weight loss goal. However, including at least brisk exercises in the schedule is very important for good health.

So, you would be required to make certain changes in your lifestyle in all three areas if you want to get the best results from intermittent fasting.

As a fast recap:

You would need to make changes in your eating patterns. You will have to follow strict eating and fasting windows. You will also have to reduce the number of meals consumed in a day.

Including healthy food items in your meals is always very helpful. You will be able to remain much healthier, and your weight would also go fast if you stop consuming fast food, processed items, fried food, and other such things. However, you can eat practically most of the things once in a while responsibly.

Exercise is important for keeping the body healthy, and it also helps in your weight loss journey. Dedicating some time to exercise every day would be very helpful.

Chapter 13:
Delicious And Easy 16:8 Method Recipes

As our final gift to you, we're going to show you how to recreate some delicious recipes which you can easily incorporate into your 16:8 eating plan. No more being hungry, no more restrictions, these recipes are delicious, easy to make, and they won't break the bank either!

For most of the receipts, you won't need any specific, or out of the ordinary cooking equipment. You will, however, need some food weighing scales, and tablespoon and teaspoons, as well as cups. These will help you weigh out the ingredients correctly, and therefore avoid you adding too much of something and either ruining the recipe, so it doesn't work out correctly, or taking the health side of the recipe too far to one side and making it unhealthy!

We're not going to give you specific meal names, e.g. breakfast, lunch, or dinner, you might not eat breakfast, and you might decide to start eating at lunchtime! Intermittent fasting overall is about choice, so these recipes are going to be varied in terms of their bulk and content, so you can choose when you want to make them. Some can also be made ahead of time and placed in the freezer - again, intermittent fasting is designed to fit in with your lifestyle, so why not make batches and then defrost them when you plan to enjoy them, perhaps after work or after a busy day doing whatever it is you do!

You'll also notice that our recipes come complete with macros, and these are the measurements of nutrition within each recipe. For instance, how many calories, how much carb content, protein, fat, etc. This will help you choose which meals to make on specific days, so that you don't go too calorie-heavy, or otherwise.

No more chat let's get down to business!

Chicken, Vegetable and Pesto Stir-fry

Servings: 4

Preparation time: 10 mins

Cooking time: 20 mins

Nutrition:

Calories 434

Carbs 18.5g

Fat 20g

Protein 8g

Ingredients

2 tbsps olive oil

6 boneless and skinless chicken thighs

2 sun-dried tomatoes, chopped roughly

4 asparagus spears

2 tbsps basil peso

8 cherry tomatoes, halved

Method:

Preheat your stove to a medium heat

Take a large skillet pan and add the olive oil, allowing it to heat up

Once hot, add the chicken to the pan and sprinkle salt over the top

Take half of the sun-dried tomatoes and add them to the pan

Cook the contents of the pan for around 10 minutes, making sure you turn the chicken over every so often

Once the chicken is cooked, take it out of the pan along with the tomatoes, but leave the oil inside

Now, add the asparagus to the pan and add a little salt

Add the rest of the sun-dried tomatoes to the pan also and cook for another 10 minutes

Once cooked, place onto a serving plate

Put the chicken back into the pan and stir in the pesto, cooking for a couple of minutes, ensuring the chicken is extremely hot

Place the chicken onto the serving plate

Serve with the cherry tomatoes on the side

Homemade Turkey Burger And Relish

Servings: 4

Preparation time: 10 mins

Cooking time: 20 mins

Nutrition:

Calories 258
Carbs 10g
Fat 13g

Protein 3g

Ingredients:

2lb ground turkey, made into four patties

1 onion, finely chopped

1 red bell pepper, chopped up finely

3 cups red cabbage, chopped or shredded

1 tbsp olive oil

0.25 cup balsamic vinegar

0.25 tsp garlic salt

4 lettuce leaves, large if possible

Method:

Take a large skillet pan and place over a medium heat

Add the olive oil and allow it to reach temperature

Add the onion, red cabbage, and the pepper to the pan and cook until everything has softened

Now add the balsamic vinegar and the garlic salt and combine everything together, letting it simmer for a few minutes until the contents have caramelized from the vinegar

Remove the contents of the pan and set aside to cool

Take your turkey patties and season with salt and pepper

Cook your patties for around 4 minutes on each side in either a pan or under the grill

Once cooked, transfer each patty onto a lettuce leaf and add some of the relishes on top

Homemade Tuna Fish Cakes With Lemon Sauce

Servings: 1

Preparation time: 10 mins

Cooking time: 20 mins

Macros per serving (2 cakes are one serving):

Calories 280

Carbs 14g

Fat 11g

Protein 4g

Ingredients:

For the tuna cakes:

Half a zucchini, grated

1 can of drained tuna

2 tbsp oats

2 tbsp cheese of your choice, shredded

1 egg

0.24 tsp garlic salt

0.25 tsp dill

0.25 tsp onion powder

For the sauce:

2 tbsp yogurt, Greek-style is best

1 tsp juice of a lemon

0.25 tsp dill

0.25 tsp garlic salt

Method:

Take a piece of cheesecloth, or similar and place the grated zucchini inside, twisting so that all the liquid comes out

In a medium bowl, place the drained zucchini inside and add the tuna, oats, shredded cheese, the garlic salt, dill, onion powder, pepper, and the egg, combining everything together well

Take a large frying pan and add a little olive oil, or cooking spray if you prefer

Take half of the mixture and form a ball, before flattening it into a fish cake style, repeating with the other half

Place the cakes into the frying pan, cooking over medium heat for around 6 minutes on each side

Meanwhile, combine the sauce ingredients into a small mixing bowl and ensure they are mixed together well

Once the fish cakes are cooked place them on a serving plate and allow to cool just slightly

Add a spoonful of the sauce on top and enjoy!

Healthy Breakfast Burritos

Servings: 4

Preparation time: 5 mins

Cooking time: 10 mins

Nutrition:

Calories 352

Carbs 22g

Fat 20g

Protein 8g

Ingredients

8 eggs

1 tbsp milk

1 tbsp garlic, minced

1 red pepper, minced

Half an onion, red if possible, minced

4 slices of bacon, cooked

Salt

Pepper

4 tortilla wraps (multi-grain or wholegrain)

A little cheese (optional)

Method:

Take a medium-sized saucepan and heat over a medium heat

Add the garlic and cook for a couple of minutes, until fragrant

Whisk the eggs with the milk and place to one side

Add the pepper and onion to the pan and allow to cook for a couple
more minutes,

Add the eggs to the pan and cook for 4 minutes

Once cooked, add a quarter of the egg mixture onto each tortilla wrap
and add one piece of the bacon on top

You can add cheese if you want, although it isn't necessary

Wrap up and enjoy!

Delicious Egg Casserole

Servings: 8

Preparation time: 10 mins

Cooking time: 30 mins

Nutrition:

Calories 370

Carbs 23g

Fat 20g

Protein 24g

Ingredients:

4.5 cups brown bread, cut into cubes

2 cups cheese, shredded

10 eggs, beaten

0.25-pint milk

1 tsp dry mustard

1 tsp salt

0/25 tsp onion powder

8 slices bacon, cooked and crumbled up

0.5 cup mushrooms, chopped

Method:

Preheat your oven to 325C

Take a baking dish, around 13 inches in size and spray it with some cooking spray, to avoid sticking

Take the cubed pieces of bread and lay them in the bottom of the baking dish, evenly, so that the bottom is totally covered over

Add the cheese on the top, in one even layer

Take a separate mixing bowl and combine the milk, mustard, eggs, pepper, onion powder and the salt until completely mixed together

Add the mixture over the top of the bread and the cheese evenly

Now add the bacon and mushrooms on top, again making sure to stick to an even layer

Place the baking dish in the oven for half an hour. You will know when it is finished because it will have turned a wonderful golden brown

Remove from the oven and place to one side to cool for ten minutes

Cut into slices and serve

Chicken Cobb Salad, With a BBQ Twist

Servings: 1

Preparation time: 10 mins

Cooking time: 25 mins

Nutrition:

Calories 280

Carbs 19g

Fat 9.5g

Protein 27.5g

Ingredients:

3oz chicken breast, no bones, and no skin

2 tbsp BBQ sauce

2 slices bacon, chopped into small pieces

1.5 cups of romaine lettuce, chopped

0.25 cups cherry tomatoes, chopped

0.25 avocado, chopped

1 boiled egg, chopped

Method:

Preheat your oven to 350C

Take the chicken and brush it with 1 tbsp of the BBQ sauce

Take a baking dish and spray with a little cooking spray

Place the chicken inside the baking dish and place into the oven for 25 minutes, or until the chicken is completely cooked through

Whilst the chicken is cooking, cook your bacon according to your preference and chop up once cooked

Take a serving bowl and place your romaine lettuce inside, arranging carefully

Add the chicken and bacon once cooked, as well as the egg, tomatoes, and the avocado

Drizzle the rest of the BBQ sauce over the top and enjoy whilst still warm

Hearty Quinoa And Carrot Soup

Servings: 4

Preparation time: 10 mins

Cooking time: 50 mins

Nutrition:

Calories 280

Carbs 44g

Fat 7g

Protein 9g

Ingredients:

1 tbsp coconut oil

1 medium onion, chopped

1 small shallot, chopped very finely

1 tsp garlic, minced

1 tsp thyme, fresh is best in this case

3 sage leaves, chopped. Again, go for fresh if you can

1 tsp cumin

0.25 tsp turmeric

A little black pepper, according to your preferences

1lb carrots, chopped

0.5lb parsnips, chopped

0.25 cup quinoa, uncooked and ensure it is rinsed out and drained thoroughly

5 cups broth, a vegetable broth is best, or you can use simple water

Method:

For this recipe, you will need a large saucepan or stockpot

Add the coconut oil and place over a medium heat

Once hot, add the garlic, onion, and the shallot and cook for around 6 minutes

Add the cumin, turmeric, thyme, and the sage, with the pepper and combine well

Now add the parsnips and the carrots and stir once more

Add the quinoa and stir again

Add the broth or the water and allow the mixture to boil

Once the pan boils, turn the heat down to a simmer

Cook for 30-40 minutes, until everything is soft and cooked through

Take the pan from the heat and place it one side for around 5 minutes, until it has cooked down

You will now need an immersion or hand blender, so you can blend up the cup until it is smooth

Serve whilst still warm

Warming Lamb Stew

Servings: 4

Preparation time: 15 mins

Cooking time: 1 hour 30 mins

Nutrition:

Calories 343

Carbs 30g

Fat 9g

Protein 28.5g

Ingredients:

2 tsp olive oil, extra virgin is best

1lb lamb, make sure it is as lean as you can get it, and cut into cubes

A little salt

A little pepper

1 large onion, chopped

1 celery stalk, chopped

2 garlic cloves, chopped

2 carrots, cut into small pieces

1.5 tsp oregano

2 cups broth, chicken broth works best here but you can use vegetable also

0.25 cup red wine, the dry version works well

1 x 15oz can of tomato sauce, the smoother the better

1 tsp zest from a lemon

0.5 tsp cinnamon

1 sweet potato, chopped

1 lemon, chopped

Method:

You will need a Dutch oven for this recipe, and you need to add the oil and set to a medium to high heat

Once heated up, add the meat and add a little salt and pepper to your taste

Sear the lamb on both sides

Now, add the celery and the onion and cook for around 4 minutes, until soft

Add the garlic and cook for half a minute

Add the oregano and combine well, and then add the carrots, stirring all the while for another half a minute

Add the wine, the broth, the tomato sauce, the lemon zest, and the cinnamon and combine everything well

Add the sweet potato and the lemon and combine once more

Allow the mixture to reach the boiling point and then turn the heat down to a lower temperature, covering over and allowing to simmer

Cook until the vegetables are soft, and the lamb is totally cooked, for between 80-90 minutes

You may need to add more salt and pepper, according to your personal preferences

Chapter 14:
Extra Tips to Get the Most Out of Intermittent Fasting

If you have followed through up until this point, then you should know by now just how beneficial intermittent fasting can be. You might have already started to implement the strategies and recipes that I have shared with you. If so, then good for you. You are on your way to a better and healthier life, a lower body weight, a better body composition, and let's not forget a reduced risk of many diseases.

Before we finish off however, I do have a few final tips that I would like to share with you. The information I have provided here is already invaluable because it will put you on the right path to lose weight successfully through both diet and the intermittent fasting program. But what I am about to share with you will ultimately help to speed up your results and give you an even greater goal to look forward to.

Adjust your diet plan as you go

Even after that, you may continue with the program in order to experience more benefits, such as reduced body weight and to gain an improvement in your overall health.

Now, at the same time, I do want to note that following one single plan over an extended period of time will often not offer you the best results that you could achieve through intermittent fasting.

The thing is every person is different; you are unique. For this reason, a specific meal plan that works for you will likely not be ideal for every single person.

Sure, you are not a dietician with years of experience in the industry, which really does make it somewhat harder for you to develop an appropriate diet plan that will suit you and help you achieve the goals you are striving toward. This, however, does not necessarily mean that it will be impossible for you to make simple adjustments in order to reach those weight loss goals.

Here's an example: you follow the diet plan that I have offered here and prepare the specific meals that I have provided you with. Even though you implement these meal plans every day and you avoid binge eating, you find that you are not losing a lot of weight. In this case, there might not be an appropriate caloric deficit in your weight management plan.

If this is the case with you, then it means you will need to adjust your diet to reduce your daily caloric intake. This will essentially improve your caloric deficit and ensure you can lose weight more effectively through your intermittent fasting weight loss plan.

Don't overlook the importance of exercise in a weight loss strategy

I have seen a lot of people start with an intermittent fasting plan and end up complaining that the program is not working for them. The same person would then tell me that they do not have a very physical lifestyle.

You should have already read the topic where I explained how intermittent fasting is used for weight loss, so you should understand that without expending calories each day, you won't be able to lose that excess fat that has accumulated inside your body.

Expending calories mean being physically active. Unfortunately, quite a large percentage of the worldwide population are living sedentary lifestyles. With a sedentary lifestyle, you are really "paving the way" for weight gain. If you are not physically active, you won't be able to burn an adequate number of calories each day for weight loss to be possible in the first place.

Thus, when you decide to follow my intermittent fasting weight loss and meal plan, then you should be sure to also include an appropriate exercise plan. Make sure you are physically active according to the prescribed standards. At a minimum, you should be physically active on a few days each week.

The more you exercise, the more calories you will burn, of course. At the same time, you should be sure not to overdo things in terms of physical activity. There really is no use in causing yourself injury due to overtraining, this will only lead to temporary disability and will make training harder for the next few days (sometimes weeks or months, if you suffer a more serious injury).

It is best to create a balanced exercise plan for yourself and then test it out. Listen to your body and understand when you are pushing yourself too hard, as well as when you have some extra capacity available to up your game at the gym.

You will have to take your daily calorie consumption into account here. This data will definitely come in handy. Calculate an appropriate exercise plan that will ensure that your daily caloric expenditure through physical exercise will reach past your daily caloric intake.

Deal with hunger pangs like a boss

Let's tackle a topic that you will likely face. Hunger pangs are something that we all experience when we first start out with an intermittent fasting plan. You suddenly have to get your body adjusted to an entirely new way of eating. No longer do you get up in the morning and cook some eggs and bacon. You have to get up and drink water, or perhaps have a cup of coffee, but you'll have to wait until the afternoon before you get to have your first meal.

So the question now is, should you give in to the temptation that you will be experiencing, especially during those first few days? Or should you implement an appropriate strategy to help you better cope with these hunger pangs and the cravings that you are going to experience?

There are different strategies that you can use to cope with your cravings. One would be to drink a glass of water if you feel hungry and you feel those cravings building up. This is an effective strategy for lots of people, but not for everyone, of course. If you find that plain water or even filtered water does not work well for you, then I suggest you try some carbonated water. Be sure not to opt for carbonated water with added sweetening agents, as these are loaded with carbs. Rather, just opt for plain sparkling water. The carbonation in the water can help to make you feel full for a while to ensure you can make it to your eating window without giving in to your temptations.

It is important that you are patient and practice self-control when cravings start building up. Giving in to these cravings should not be considered okay now-and-then, as this will break the fasting window and it will yield less effective results compared to ensuring you last until you are inside of your feeding window.

Avoid eating these foods

With intermittent fasting, a lot of people tend to follow their usual eating habits in terms of the specific foods that they put on their plate during each meal, expecting that they will lose weight just because they have fasted during the morning, night, and a part of the afternoon.

While intermittent fasting may help to improve metabolism and support digestive function that will ultimately improve your ability to lose weight, the food you eat still counts. As you might have noted, the meal plans that I shared with you is generally combine a range of healthy foods in order to ensure you get the nutrients you need without loading up on too many carbs. I did include a lot of delicious options that you can try out.

Just as there are a lot of foods that you can surely include in your diet to help you lose that extra weight that is causing you concern, there are also some foods that you should always try to avoid if your goal is to lose weight.

Below, I would like to share some of the most important foods that you should try to exclude from your diet in order to improve the results you are able to achieve when you implement the recipes and meal plans I have provided.

- Fried foods, of course, are at the top of my list. There is no doubt that fried foods are one particularly common reason why the world is so obese. Millions of people eat fried foods as much as every day. This does not only cause them to gain weight, but also to experience a rise in cholesterol levels, be at a higher risk of heart disease, and more.

- Fast foods, along with fried foods, since most chains that offer fast foods tend to deep-fry their food in the worst types of oil and fat to make them more "tasty" for the general public. Unfortunately, this also adds more fat to your belly, thighs, arms, and other areas of your body.

- Corn is another food that really isn't the best choice for people who are trying to lose weight. Sure, it is not an unhealthy food, but consider the fact that this is a type of grain that is relatively high in sugar. The sugar spike experienced when you eat corn leads to the release of insulin, triggering inflammation and taking you one step closer to the dreadful complications of insulin resistance.

In addition to all of these, be sure to be wary of added sugars in everything you eat. For example, if you visit your local supermarket and grab a health bar to use as the food to break your fast, the fact that the word "healthy" appears on the bar does not necessarily mean it is truly healthy.

Always look at the ingredients of what you buy and what you will be putting into your body. Making your own healthy energy bars at home might be a better solution as well.

Conclusion

Congratulations on saying NO to ill health, stubborn weight gain, depression, dementia and premature ageing, and a loud NO to the idea that we cannot naturally heal our bodies and minds! When I first sat down to write this guide to understand and use the secrets of intermittent fasting, to people like you: those who are not satisfied with the current state of affairs, which they had been told and did not do that. They are ready to let go of their desire for good health, vitality, physical fitness, clarity of mind and longevity just because conventional medicine and nutrition tells them that this is impossible. Continuing your journey to achieve liveliness and well-being for life, remember that you are travelling through an old, proven form of prosperity. I urge you to use this as a guide. When people ask about the use of intermittent fasting, you will not only be able to point to visible changes in your body, appearance and energy levels, but you have all the scientific evidence at hand to prove that the old method works! Live and heal! These days it works just as well as centuries ago! Finally, I wish you all the best on your journey to restore, rejuvenate and protect every cell in your body and mind. This is handy for use with different types of intermittent fasting, which we cover in this guide! Go luck and good health!